Introduction

Angina and heart attacks kill more men in the UK than any other single disease, and six times more women than breast cancer. The cause of these conditions is a disease of the coronary arteries, the vital blood vessels only a few millimetres in diameter that supply blood to the heart muscle. The coronary arteries in patients with angina become gradually clogged with fat, and if they block completely they cause a heart attack. Doctors call this process coronary heart disease, or CHD for short.

Coronary heart disease has become more common all over the western world in the last 50 years, and most people will know a friend or a relative who has had a heart attack, often without warning. Medical research has discovered some of the important factors responsible for CHD and we now know many ways by which we can prevent it happening in people at risk. This book gives an account of how and why this disease occurs and what we can do about it.

What's in a name?

There are several terms used to describe coronary disease and its effects on the heart. Coronary heart disease is the one used in this book, but others that you may hear doctors use are shown in the box.

Abbreviation	Name	What is it?
CAD	Coronary artery disease	Disease of the coronary arteries themselves
IHD	Ischaemic heart disease	Narrowing of the blood vessels results in ischaemia, that is, lack of blood supply to the heart muscle
MI	Myocardial infarction, coronary thrombosis, heart attack	Death of an area of heart muscle as a result of blockage in blood supply

Coronary artery disease can cause a number of different problems for the heart, all the result of insufficient oxygen reaching the heart muscle. The following are the most common.

Angina

A pain in the chest that comes on typically when exercising; this can include everyday physical effort, not just activities such as aerobics or jogging! The pain gets better when you rest.

Understanding
Angina and Heart Attacks

Dr Chris Davidson

Published by Family Doctor Publications Limited
in association with the British Medical Association

IMPORTANT

This book is intended not as a substitute for personal
medical advice but as a supplement to that advice for
the patient who wishes to understand more about his
or her condition.

Before taking any form of treatment
YOU SHOULD ALWAYS CONSULT YOUR MEDICAL
PRACTITIONER.

In particular (without limit) you should note that
advances in medical science occur rapidly and some
information about drugs and treatment contained in this
booklet may very soon be out of date.

© Family Doctor Publications 1998–2006
Updated 2000, 2002, 2003, 2004, 2006

Family Doctor Publications, PO Box 4664, Poole, Dorset BH15 1NN

ISBN: 1 903474 22 1

Contents

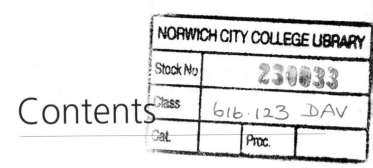

Introduction 1

What goes wrong? 12

Causes of CHD – why me? 33

Recognising the symptoms 45

Tests for CHD 54

Treating angina 65

Treating a heart attack 81

Getting over a heart attack 92

Look after your heart 98

Useful addresses 115

Index 125

Your pages 135

About the author

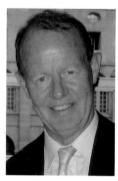

Dr Chris Davidson is a cardiologist at Brighton, and was previously a Consultant Physician at Rochdale. He has had extensive experience in coronary heart disease and high blood pressure, and is currently chairman of the Committee on Cardiac Rehabilitation of the British Heart Foundation.

Heart attack (myocardial infarction or MI)
Life-threatening chest pain when the artery blocks completely, resulting in damage to an area of heart muscle.

Other conditions that are often the result of coronary heart disease include the following.

Heart failure
The heart muscle is so damaged that it cannot pump enough blood to the rest of the body, leading to breathlessness and fluid retention.

Irregularities of heart rhythm (arrhythmias)
Irregular beats can cause palpitations but are sometimes serious enough to stop the heart beating altogether.

Other causes of heart problems
Not all heart disease is coronary artery disease, but it is far and away the most common cause in the UK. Other heart problems include the following.

Congenital heart disease
Abnormalities of the heart that are present at birth, such as a hole in the heart.

Cardiomyopathies
Diseases that damage the heart muscle directly rather than the coronary arteries.

Valvular heart disease
Damage to any of the four valves that control blood flow in the heart.

Deaths by cause, men and women under 75

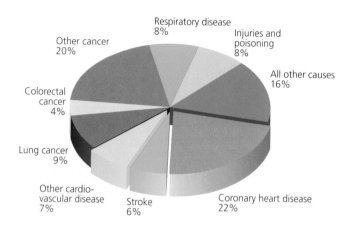

UK men

Respiratory disease 8%

Injuries and poisoning 8%

Other cancer 20%

All other causes 16%

Colorectal cancer 4%

Lung cancer 9%

Other cardio-vascular disease 7%

Stroke 6%

Coronary heart disease 22%

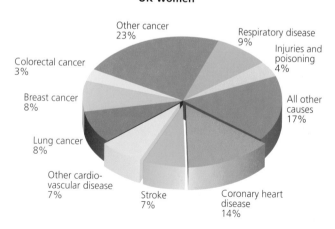

UK women

Other cancer 23%

Respiratory disease 9%

Injuries and poisoning 4%

Colorectal cancer 3%

Breast cancer 8%

All other causes 17%

Lung cancer 8%

Other cardio-vascular disease 7%

Stroke 7%

Coronary heart disease 14%

Source: British Heart Foundation Statistics Database.

Who gets heart disease?

The number of people who get CHD varies enormously from one country to another. We are all used to the idea that certain diseases are more common in one country than another, yet we don't usually see our own country in the same way. But if we were looking down on the Earth from another planet we would be as struck by the very high rates of heart disease in the British Isles as we might be by malaria in the tropics.

A disease of affluence

In general, CHD is a disease of affluence and is much less common in developing countries such as Africa. It is most common in northern Europe, North America and Australasia. It does seem to be related in some way to lifestyle, because when people move from the developing countries to a more affluent culture they get CHD much more often than they would have done

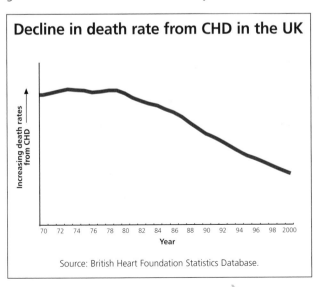

Source: British Heart Foundation Statistics Database.

Death rate from CHD by area in the UK

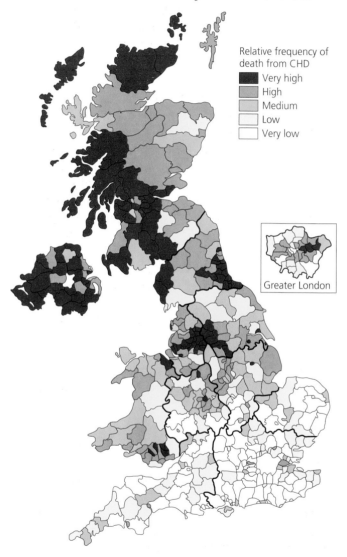

Relative frequency of
death from CHD

- Very high
- High
- Medium
- Low
- Very low

Greater London

Source: British Heart Foundation Statistics Database.

at home. This is particularly noticeable among immigrants from the Indian subcontinent who come to the UK and who are then even more likely to develop CHD than people who were born here.

Regional variations

Within Europe there are major differences between countries and even within one country. In southern Europe, CHD is generally much less common than in the UK and Scandinavia – and this may be one of the reasons for the popularity of the Mediterranean diet at present. Many people believe that this way of eating – with lots of fresh vegetables, salad, fruit and fish and relatively little red meat or dairy produce – can help protect against heart disease (more about this on pages 104–7).

In the UK itself there are also large variations between regions; the highest rates are in what were the old areas of industrialisation – northern England, Scotland, Wales and Northern Ireland.

When was CHD first recognised?

Although descriptions of CHD date back to the classical world, it was not recognised to be a common disease until after World War II. The rate of heart disease, particularly among young men, rose alarmingly. It peaked in the USA and Australia in 1970s and in the UK in the mid-1980s and has been falling steadily ever since. Unfortunately, rates of CHD are rising rapidly in eastern Europe, with countries such as Russia and the Baltic states now heading the league table. There are also worrying trends in Asia where affluence has brought with it a sharp rise in CHD.

Variations in CHD across Europe

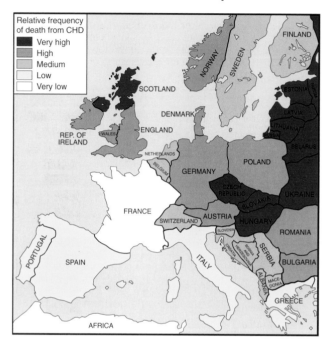

In spite of the improvements in the UK in recent years, CHD remains a serious public health problem. It is much more common in elderly people and four times more common in men than in premenopausal women (women who have not yet had their last menstrual cycle). In young men it is the most common cause of death after accidents.

What are the probable causes of CHD?

Why is CHD so common in the UK? No one knows for sure, but diet, smoking, lack of exercise and social deprivation seem likely culprits. Of course poverty, lack

Comparative death rate from CHD by country

CHD is generally higher in the more affluent countries than in developing nations. The rates are particularly high in the old Eastern bloc nations. The table below shows the comparative death rates for men and women in a selection of countries.

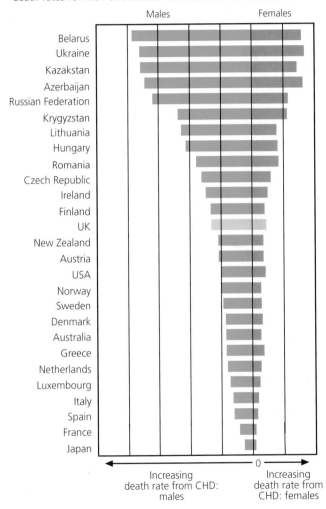

of exercise and smoking also occur in other countries where the risk of CHD is much lower, and this is why there is so much focus on the British diet as a potential cause. In the UK there are particular concerns at the moment about the rising numbers of people who are overweight, even as children, and unless this is corrected we may see the risk of CHD increasing again.

New treatments for CHD

The last 10 years have seen enormous advances in the treatment of CHD. There are new drugs, such as the 'clot busters' used after a heart attack, better drugs for angina and powerful cholesterol-lowering drugs, to name just a few. And we have come to understand the value of some of the older drugs such as beta blockers and aspirin. Not only can these help in relieving symptoms such as pain, but they can also slow down or even reverse some of the changes seen in the disease.

The biggest advances, however, have been in the use of surgery and angioplasty. Bypass surgery (CABG – often pronounced as 'cabbage'! – which stands for coronary artery bypass graft) can transform the life of an angina sufferer and can reduce the risk of further heart attacks.

Angioplasty – a technique in which tiny balloons are used to stretch narrowed or blocked arteries – can also be very effective, especially now that fine wire stents (or internal supports) are used to keep the arteries open.

This is all good news for anyone who has already developed heart trouble but our priority as a country should be to tackle the underlying reasons why CHD is so common and try to stop so many people getting it in the first place.

KEY POINTS

- CHD is still one of the most common causes of death in the UK for both men and women

- There was an epidemic of CHD in the twentieth century, which is now declining in the UK but rising in countries in eastern Europe

- New treatments, including bypass surgery, have helped a lot, but prevention remains better than cure

What goes wrong?

How your heart works

The heart is a muscular pump in the chest that is constantly working, pumping blood around your body, day and night, from cradle to grave. It contracts and relaxes 100,000 times a day, and needs a good blood supply of its own – one provided by the coronary arteries.

The basic function of the heart is to pump red blood, which is rich in oxygen and nutrients, through large arteries to the rest of the body. When the oxygen has been taken up by muscles and other tissues, veins carry the blood (now blue and deoxygenated) back to the heart.

There are two sides to the heart, each of which acts as a separate pump. The two halves are subdivided into two chambers, four in all. The upper ones, the atria, act as collecting reservoirs and the lower ones, the ventricles, contract to pump the blood on. The right side of the heart receives blood from veins draining the whole body and pumps it through the lungs so that it can pick up oxygen, changing from

Cardiovascular system

Diagram showing the heart and circulation with veins (blue) draining the blood back to the heart where it is pumped to the lungs and back to the rest of the body through the arteries (red). Larger blood vessels branch into smaller and smaller ones and then to tiny networks of blood vessels known as capillaries, where oxygen and nutrients are passed from the blood into the surrounding cells.

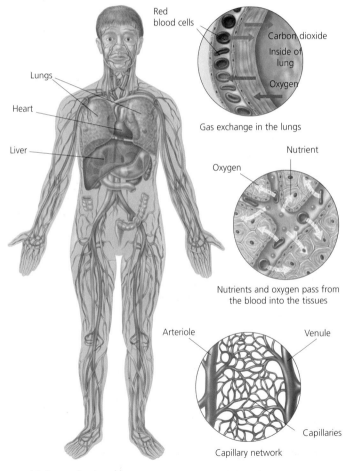

Red blood cells

Carbon dioxide

Inside of lung

Oxygen

Gas exchange in the lungs

Lungs

Heart

Liver

Nutrient

Oxygen

Nutrients and oxygen pass from the blood into the tissues

Arteriole

Venule

Capillaries

Capillary network

Arteries = red, veins = blue

How blood circulates around the body

Deoxygenated blood (blue) from the body organs and tissues enters the right-hand side of the heart and is pumped through the lungs where it takes up oxygen. This oxygenated blood (red) then re-enters the left-hand side of the heart and is pumped out to the body.

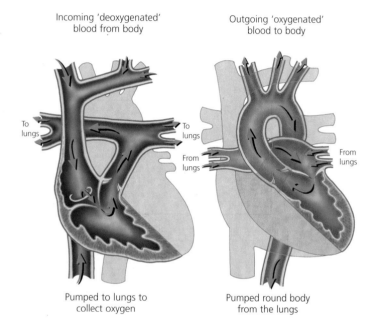

Incoming 'deoxygenated' blood from body

Outgoing 'oxygenated' blood to body

To lungs

To lungs

From lungs

From lungs

Pumped to lungs to collect oxygen

Pumped round body from the lungs

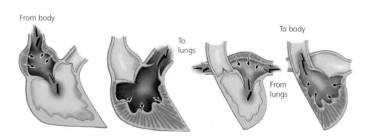

From body

To lungs

To body

From lungs

Right heart

Left heart

The internal structure of the heart

This diagram shows the four chambers of the heart which work together in two pairs in a rhythmic cycle. A valve at the exit of each chamber prevents blood from flowing backwards in the wrong direction.

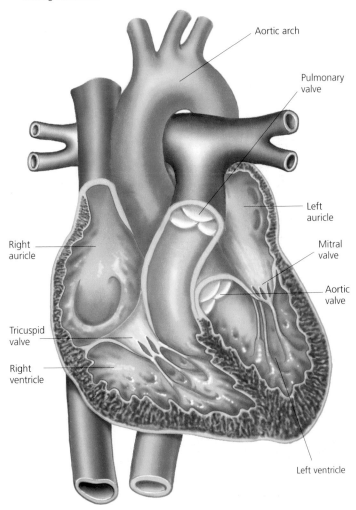

Aortic arch

Pulmonary valve

Left auricle

Right auricle

Mitral valve

Aortic valve

Tricuspid valve

Right ventricle

Left ventricle

blue to red. The left side then collects blood returning from the lungs and pumps it round the body to the tissues that need oxygen.

In order to reach all the different organs and muscles, blood has to be pumped at high pressure, as you will certainly know if you have ever cut an artery – the blood spurts everywhere! To do this heart muscle is very strong and, unlike other muscles, it never becomes fatigued. Heart muscle, therefore, is crucially dependent on a reliable blood supply and this is provided by the coronary arteries and their branches.

The coronary arteries

The coronary arteries come off the aorta – the main blood vessel from the heart – just as it leaves the pumping chamber, the left ventricle, so they are the first arteries to receive blood high in oxygen. The two arteries, the right and the left, are relatively small (three to four millimetres in diameter). They pass over the surface of the heart, meeting each other at the back almost forming a circle. When this pattern of blood vessels was first seen by the ancients, they thought it looked like a crown and so they used the Latin name (*corona*) that we have today – the coronary arteries.

The left coronary artery has two main branches, called the anterior descending and the circumflex, which in turn have other branches of their own. It supplies most of the left ventricle which is the more muscular of the two ventricles because it has to pump blood around the whole of the body. The right coronary artery is usually smaller and supplies the underside of the heart and the right ventricle, the chamber that pumps blood to the lungs.

The blood supply to the heart

The right and left coronary arteries arise from the beginning of the aortic arch. These two arteries then branch into smaller vessels that supply oxygenated blood to the muscles of the heart.

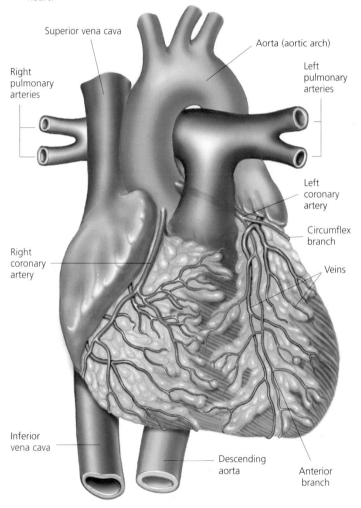

Superior vena cava

Aorta (aortic arch)

Right pulmonary arteries

Left pulmonary arteries

Left coronary artery

Circumflex branch

Right coronary artery

Veins

Inferior vena cava

Descending aorta

Anterior branch

What happens to the coronary arteries in CHD?

In CHD, the coronary arteries become narrowed (rather like a water pipe becomes 'furred up' in a hard water area), and the heart muscle becomes starved of the blood and oxygen that it needs. At rest this may not matter, but if the heart tries to work harder than normal – for example, if you walk up stairs – the blood supply may be insufficient and you get a pain in your chest (see 'Angina' on page 46). If you rest for a few minutes, the pain usually goes away. If the coronary artery is blocked completely by a blood clot, the area of the heart muscle that it supplies will die (see 'Heart attack' on page 47).

Atheroma

Hardening of the arteries, atheroma and atherosclerosis are all the same thing. When you are born, your blood vessels are flexible and elastic and the blood can flow through them with ease. Early in adult life, however, fat deposits can start to form on the walls of the arteries. They gradually build up, forming lumps that protrude into the middle of the artery and reduce blood flow.

The extent of these changes and the rate at which they occur are affected by the level of the fats in the blood (technically called lipids), especially one called low-density lipoprotein-cholesterol, or LDL-cholesterol for short (see page 99). People who have high blood levels of LDL-cholesterol are more likely to develop severe atheroma, but some changes may be present in all of us by the time we reach middle age.

The patches of atheroma are called plaques and, as they grow, they thicken and weaken the wall of the artery and progressively reduce blood flow. This process

The process of atheroma

Atheroma is the process by which fat is deposited on the inside walls of blood vessels. The deposits can grow to such extent that they restrict blood flow.

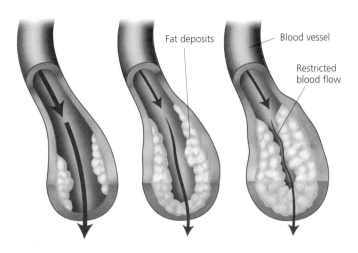

Fat deposits

Blood vessel

Restricted blood flow

can affect any part of the body, so that in the arteries to the brain atheroma can lead to a stroke, in the trunk to an aneurysm, in the limb to gangrene and in the heart to a heart attack.

What arteries are affected?

The process of hardening of the arteries is curiously patchy throughout the body, and particularly so in the coronary arteries. Narrowing can occur in just one coronary artery or part of one, or it can affect the artery throughout its length. This may be important in deciding what treatment would suit you best.

In CHD, doctors often talk of one-, two- or three-vessel disease. This refers to whether the three main branches are affected – that is to say, the two main

The clinical effects of atheroma

Diagram of the body showing the sites affected and the possible effects of atheroma.

Coronary heart disease
In CHD the coronary arteries that supply the heart muscle with nutrients become narrowed and the heart muscle becomes starved of the blood that it needs

Stroke
When a blood vessel supplying vital nutrients to the brain becomes blocked, the brain cells that it supplies will die

Aneurysm
Fatty deposits in an artery can cause the artery wall to bulge and weaken. This can rupture with catastrophic consequences

Gangrene
If arteries supplying the lower half of your body become blocked, gangrene may develop

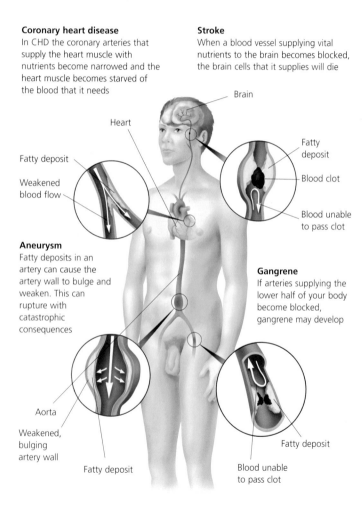

Brain

Heart

Fatty deposit

Blood clot

Blood unable to pass clot

Fatty deposit

Weakened blood flow

Aorta

Weakened, bulging artery wall

Fatty deposit

Fatty deposit

Blood unable to pass clot

branches of the left coronary artery and the right coronary artery. In general, one- or two-vessel disease may be treated with medicines or angioplasty, whereas three-vessel disease, which affects all the major coronary arteries, usually requires bypass surgery.

Thrombosis

Thrombosis is the medical term for a blood clot, and is the natural process that comes into play to stop bleeding if we injure ourselves. It is also important to stop blood clotting at the wrong time, and so we have chemicals circulating in our blood that are natural anticoagulants or blood thinners.

When we cut ourselves and a blood vessel is damaged, a whole series of chemicals is released close by, activating the blood and causing it to clot. In the case of coronary disease, a clot forms, not because of an outside injury, but as a result of damage to the lining of the artery caused by the fat that has built up there.

Normally, the lining of our arteries is smooth and there is nowhere that a clot can form. When atheroma develops the lining is no longer smooth and, where there are breaks in the surface, small cells from the blood called platelets stick to these breaks and help to seal them. Provided that the breaks are small, no harm results, but where the artery is critically narrowed even a small clot can have an important effect on blood flow. We now know that such a process is the main cause of sudden deterioration in angina – so-called unstable angina (see page 46).

In a heart attack a rather different process is probably responsible. The fatty deposit in the artery is surrounded by scar tissue caused by the cholesterol itself. This forms a fibrous cap over the top of the deposit which is much more rigid than the rest of the artery.

Any sudden stress can cause this cap to split, creating a much wider area of damage to the wall of the artery. As a result a much larger clot forms, one that usually blocks the artery altogether. Blood cannot then reach the heart muscle beyond this clot and so that section of muscle dies.

Thrombosis, then, is one of the central problems in CHD. It is the cause of most cases of sudden deterioration in angina and of most heart attacks. As we shall see, new and highly effective treatments for CHD work by removing these clots. There are complex drugs that can dissolve the clot itself in a heart attack, and simpler, but equally effective, drugs such as aspirin that can prevent a clot forming in the first place.

Heart attack

A heart attack results when the diseased coronary artery becomes completely blocked by a clot, or thrombus. The heart muscle (or myocardium) beyond the clot is suddenly starved of blood and oxygen, and becomes painful, a pain that becomes more intense as the minutes pass. Unless the clot disperses by itself, which doesn't often happen, this area of heart muscle dies within 5 to 10 minutes, resulting in a fully blown heart attack, or myocardial infarction (MI) to give it its technical name.

The actual size of the heart attack and the amount of damaged muscle depend on a number of factors. The first is the size of the artery: the bigger the artery that is blocked the bigger the area of damage. The second is that the area of damage is generally greater if other coronary arteries are also diseased. Finally, the

Coronary thrombosis

A coronary thrombosis occurs when a clot forms in the coronary arteries that supply blood to the heart muscle. In a heart attack a clot typically forms on a break in the fibrous plaque in a diseased vessel.

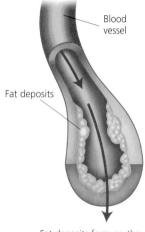

Blood vessel

Fat deposits

Fat deposits form on the walls of the artery

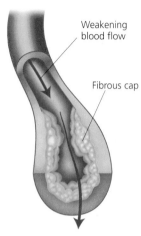

Weakening blood flow

Fibrous cap

Scar tissue forms a fibrous cap over the fat deposits

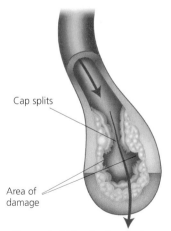

Cap splits

Area of damage

The cap is rigid and splits, creating a wider area of damage

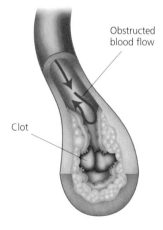

Obstructed blood flow

Clot

A large clot forms to seal the damaged area; this blocks the artery

What happens in a heart attack?

A heart attack results when one or more of the blood vessels taking oxygen to the heart muscle become blocked by a blood clot.

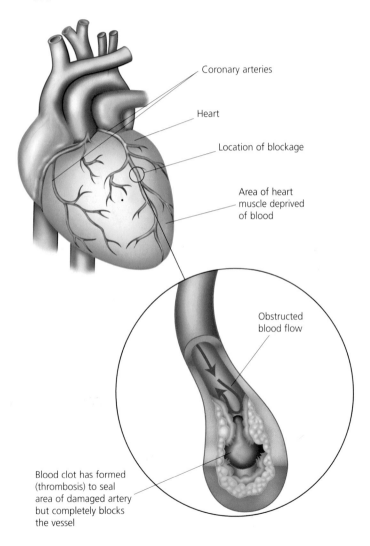

Coronary arteries

Heart

Location of blockage

Area of heart muscle deprived of blood

Obstructed blood flow

Blood clot has formed (thrombosis) to seal area of damaged artery but completely blocks the vessel

size of the heart attack depends on whether the area of muscle has developed any collateral blood supply (see page 26).

If collateral arteries have developed to supply the threatened area, the damage is much less. Regular exercise is a good stimulus to the formation of collateral vessels, which is one reason why it forms such an important part of the treatment programmes of people with CHD.

The immediate effect of the damage to the muscle, apart from pain, is that the heart no longer pumps as effectively as before, and the blood pressure may fall, leading to faintness and sweating or nausea. The other major problem in the early stages is the irregularities of heart rhythm, or cardiac arrhythmias. These arrhythmias can be life threatening and lead to a cardiac arrest. As a result, it is vital that the heart is monitored closely in the first 48 hours or so, and this is usually carried out in hospitals in cardiac care units (CCUs for short). Fortunately, arrhythmias are rare after the first two to three days, and that is when most people can go to the main ward to recover before going home.

After a heart attack, the body begins to repair the damage straight away. Cells remove the dead or damaged muscle and fibrous or scar tissue is formed, a process that takes about six to eight weeks. The scar itself is strong, but unfortunately the heart muscle that has been lost cannot be replaced and some weakening of the heart is inevitable. For many people with a small heart attack this makes very little difference to the overall performance of the heart as a pump. If a larger area of muscle is damaged, however, the heart becomes enlarged, and can no longer pump effectively, a condition we call heart failure.

Collateral circulation

When an artery is blocked the body is often able to form a network of small blood vessels to carry blood around the blockage and maintain blood flow.

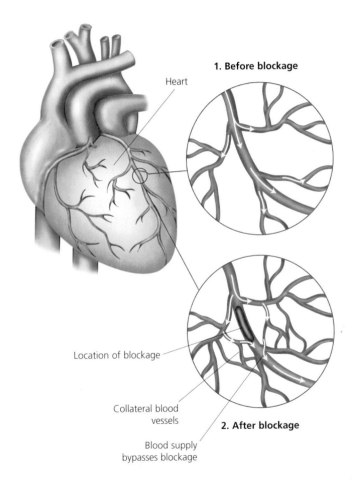

1. Before blockage

Heart

Location of blockage

Collateral blood vessels

2. After blockage

Blood supply bypasses blockage

Heart failure

Heart failure can be caused by many diseases affecting the heart, especially high blood pressure, but, in this country, CHD is probably the most common. When the heart stops pumping properly, fluid collects in the airspaces of the lungs, leading to breathlessness. Congestion of the rest of the body also leads to fluid retention, which makes the ankles and legs swell.

For many years the mainstay of treatment has been diuretics or 'water tablets', which get rid of excess fluid in the body and lungs. Now, however, we have new drugs called ACE (angiotensin-converting enzyme) inhibitors (see page 90) as well as beta blockers (see page 69) which are also highly effective in this condition.

The other result of the scarring of heart muscle is that it interferes with the electrical processes responsible for maintaining normal heart rhythm. This leads to irregularities, or cardiac arrhythmias. The most common of these is called atrial fibrillation, which is usually treated with digoxin, an old drug derived from the foxglove. Other irregularities can be treated with beta blockers and newer drugs are also now available. See the Family Doctor book *Understanding Heart Failure*.

What happens with time?

Coronary heart disease is a gradual and unpredictable condition. The fatty deposits in arteries may build up very slowly over the course of 20 or 30 years. For most of that time there are no symptoms and angina becomes a problem only when one or more of the coronary arteries narrow by more than 70 per cent and significantly affect blood flow.

Breathlessness

Breathlessness is a common symptom of heart failure.

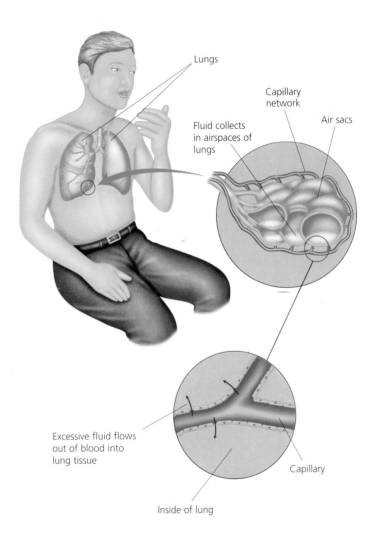

Lungs

Capillary network

Air sacs

Fluid collects in airspaces of lungs

Excessive fluid flows out of blood into lung tissue

Capillary

Inside of lung

Swollen ankles

Swollen ankles can be a symptom of heart failure.

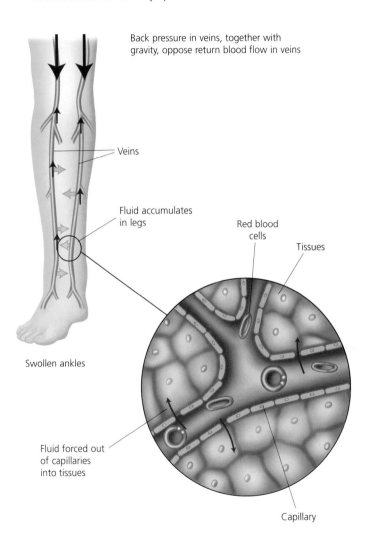

Back pressure in veins, together with gravity, oppose return blood flow in veins

Veins

Fluid accumulates in legs

Red blood cells

Tissues

Swollen ankles

Fluid forced out of capillaries into tissues

Capillary

As the process is so slow the heart can find ways of overcoming these changes by developing new blood vessels called collaterals (see page 26). The coronary arteries in effect form a network of blood vessels around the heart and, when one is narrowed, one of the other branches expands with collaterals to help the area of heart muscle affected.

Although the build-up of coronary atheroma is slow, a clot can occur at any time. People who experience only occasional angina may get a sudden worsening of their condition. Fortunately this doesn't happen very often; only about five per cent of people with angina per year experience a heart attack.

What is more worrying is the fact that a heart attack can occur 'out of the blue' in someone who has never been aware that he or she has a heart condition at all. This can happen because quite a small fatty deposit, one that causes no real problem in terms of blood flow, can suddenly split and a clot can block off the artery.

We are now beginning to understand this process rather better and there are new drugs that may prevent this happening.

Case histories
Arthur, aged 64
Three months ago, Arthur found that he was getting a pain in his chest whenever he walked up stairs or when he walked up the hill to his home, especially on cold days. Arthur's GP told him that he had angina and started him on treatment with a regular anti-anginal medicine called atenolol – Arthur now feels well again and has no symptoms.

John, aged 52

John was a keen athlete and ran marathons. His father died of a heart attack (MI) when he was 64. John had been feeling quite well, but he collapsed with chest pain and died suddenly during a 10-mile run. A postmortem examination revealed that the cause of death was a heart attack.

KEY POINTS

■ To function as a pump, heart muscle is critically dependent on the coronary arteries for a good blood supply

■ In CHD, the coronary arteries become narrowed by fatty deposits or atheroma

■ Narrowing of the coronary arteries by atheroma starves the heart muscle of oxygen and this results in the pain of angina

■ A heart attack results when a diseased coronary artery blocks completely with a clot, and the heart muscle beyond dies

■ After a heart attack the damaged muscle heals by forming a scar; provided that it is not too big complete recovery can be expected

Causes of CHD – why me?

Understanding risk factors

There does not seem to be one single cause for coronary heart disease (CHD), or at least we have not yet found one. Medical research has, however, shown that a whole range of things can make us more likely to develop CHD and these have been called risk factors. Just as a tall man is more likely to hit his head on a door frame than a small one, so people with one or more risk factors are more likely to have a heart attack than those without any. Not every tall man hits his head on a door and not every person with risk factors gets a heart attack, but the likelihood is greater.

The risk factors for CHD are divided into those that we can do something about – modifiable – and those that we cannot – non-modifiable (see table on page 34). The risk of you or me developing CHD becomes greater the more risk factors we have, and these risks multiply together. So, for example, a smoker with a high cholesterol level and high blood pressure has a

Risk factors for heart disease

Modifiable (we can change)	Non-modifiable (we cannot change)
• Smoking • Raised cholesterol • High blood pressure • Diabetes • Obesity • Stress • Lack of exercise	• Genetic factors, e.g. an inherited high cholesterol level • Gender – more men than women get CHD • Age

much higher risk than if he or she had any of these factors by themselves.

On the other hand, a high cholesterol level by itself in someone who has no other risk factors means that the risk is only increased slightly above average. This may well be nothing much to worry about if you are otherwise fit. If in doubt your doctor will be able to give you individual advice on this.

Age and gender

Heart disease, like many other diseases, becomes more common as we get older. In the UK at present, half the heart attacks occur in people over the age of 65, and the numbers are rising as the average age of the population increases.

The striking thing about CHD is that, below the age of 55, it is a much more common disease among men than women. This is because, before the menopause (the change of life when women stop menstruating), women very rarely have heart attacks. After the menopause, CHD becomes more common so that the rate among women gradually catches up with that of men, and over the age of 75 the numbers are about equal.

The exact reason why women are protected from CHD before the menopause is not known for sure but it does seem likely that this is related to hormones that disappear once menstruation stops. Unfortunately HRT (hormone replacement therapy) does not prevent heart attacks if taken after the menopause, although it may be helpful for other problems such as osteoporosis.

Family history

Doctors talk about a positive family history when one or more close relatives (parents, brothers, sisters or children) have had CHD. If your father had a heart attack below the age of 60 or your mother below the age of 65, this increases your own risk of CHD. Of course, if your parents lived to old age when heart attacks are common anyway, this is not so important.

The same also applies to brothers and sisters, although, in very large families, the fact that one member may have a heart attack could be just the result of chance.

How is it that CHD runs in families? Part of the explanation is from the genes that we inherit from our parents that may make us more liable to have high cholesterol, high blood pressure or diabetes. Part may also be the result of families living similar lifestyles – they all eat the same food and, if parents smoke, often their children do too.

If heart disease does appear to run in your family it is very useful to have check-ups from time to time with your doctor, to make sure that you have not developed high cholesterol, high blood pressure or other problems that could be treated to reduce your risk.

Diet and cholesterol

As we have already seen, atheroma is the major cause of coronary artery disease. Deposits of fat and, especially, of cholesterol, known as plaques, form in the walls of the arteries. This makes them narrower and so reduces blood flow. When plaques split, a clot forms on the damaged area, stopping the blood flow and leading to a heart attack. This whole process is more likely to happen (and to cause more damage if it does) in a person who has a high level of cholesterol in the blood.

Your genetic make-up is partly responsible for determining your cholesterol level. Some families carry genes for raised levels of blood fats. This condition is called familial hyperlipidaemia or FH for short. However, diet also plays an important part in the cholesterol levels in your blood. The more fats – particularly animal and dairy fat – that you eat, the

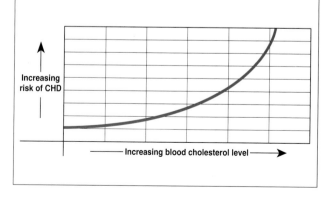

Cholesterol and higher CHD risk

The higher the level of cholesterol in your blood, the greater is your risk of developing heart disease. You can lower your cholesterol by changes in your diet, particularly by reducing your intake of animal and dairy fat.

Increasing risk of CHD

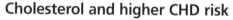

Increasing blood cholesterol level

higher your cholesterol will be and the higher your risk of CHD (see diagram on page 36). So it really is worth reducing the animal fat content in your diet (for more on this, see page 104).

See the Family Doctor book *Understanding Cholesterol* for a fuller discussion.

Smoking

Cigarette smoking is strongly linked to the risk of CHD. Chemicals in cigarette smoke are absorbed into your bloodstream from the lungs and circulate around the body, affecting every cell. These chemicals make the blood vessels narrow temporarily. They also cause blood cells called platelets to become stickier, so increasing the chance of a clot forming.

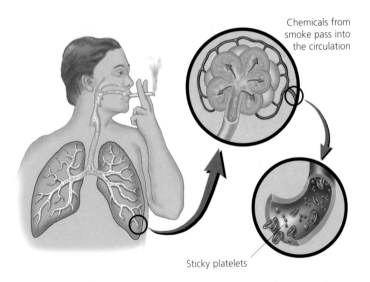

Chemicals from smoke pass into the circulation

Sticky platelets

Smoking makes blood platelets 'stickier', so increasing the likelihood of blood clots forming in the circulation.

The Framingham study

One of the first studies that linked high cholesterol with CHD was carried out after World War II in a small town near Boston, USA called Framingham. All the residents were examined at yearly intervals to see whether or not they had developed CHD. A strong link with raised cholesterol was found early on – the higher the blood cholesterol, the higher the risk of developing a heart attack. The Framingham study also showed the importance of the other risk factors such as smoking, high blood pressure and diabetes, and these risk factors have been confirmed over a follow-up period of nearly 40 years since the study first started. The study is still continuing.

Pipe and cigar smokers do not have the high risk of cigarette smokers but are still more likely to get CHD than non-smokers. The amount that you smoke also matters; the risk increases stepwise from light (fewer than 10 cigarettes per day), to moderate (10–20 cigarettes per day), to heavy smokers (more than 20 cigarettes per day).

The reason why doctors place such stress on stopping smoking is that it is the one risk factor that you can control yourself. What's more, you start to reap the benefit from the moment you stop. Although your risk of CHD may never be quite as low as that of a non-smoker, it certainly comes close to it a year or two after stopping.

Stress

Many people who have had a heart attack point to some personal stress as a cause, but it has been surprisingly difficult to prove this link scientifically. There are well-recognised trigger factors, such as sudden unexpected exercise or extreme emotional experiences, which can bring on a heart attack, but this is fairly rare. Yet at times of great civil and military stress, such as in World War II, the number of heart attacks in the civilian population actually fell.

We also think of certain personality types as having a higher risk of heart disease. Modern technology has brought with it the ability to do things in minutes that even a generation ago might have taken days. The pressure to take on more than you can manage, to set unrealistic goals, has created the idea of the type A personality. This restless individual (usually male) finds it difficult to relax, becomes increasingly tied up in work at the expense of personal relationships and is prone in

Risk factors for CHD

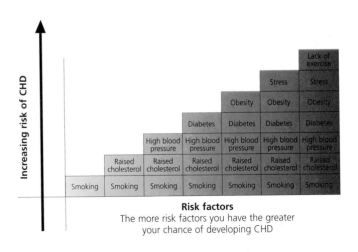

Risk factors
The more risk factors you have the greater your chance of developing CHD

the end to 'burn-out'. He is said to have double the risk of CHD compared with the 'laid-back' type B personality.

This theory linking CHD and the stressful personality was once very fashionable, and a lot of effort was put in to persuade people who had worked hard all their lives to relax. Modern research has failed to confirm these earlier findings and, although a major illness of any kind is a good time to take stock of priorities in life, attempts to make major changes in behaviour are probably of little benefit.

Other diseases linked to CHD

Two common and important diseases are associated with a higher than average risk of CHD:

- high blood pressure (BP)

- diabetes.

High blood pressure
What is blood pressure?

The term 'blood pressure' means the pressure in the arteries taking blood from the heart to the rest of the body. High blood pressure causes stresses on the heart and circulation, and most people are aware that it causes strokes. However, in the UK high blood pressure is responsible for more heart attacks than strokes, probably because of the high cholesterol levels present in individuals in this country. Treatment of high blood pressure will reduce the risk of both heart attack and stroke.

How is blood pressure measured?

Blood pressure is usually measured in the upper arm. With each beat of the heart, the blood pressure rises to a high point (systolic pressure) and then falls to a low point between beats (diastolic pressure). This pressure is measured in millimetres of mercury (mmHg). An average healthy person's blood pressure at rest is around 120/70, said as 120 over 70. A resting pressure of 140/90 is borderline, whereas 150/100 is definitely raised.

140

Systolic pressure
The pressure produced in the circulation when the heart contracts

90

Diastolic pressure
The pressure in the circulation between heartbeats

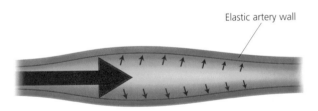

Elastic artery wall

Blood pressure wave from beat of heart

Greater pressure

Lower pressure

Blood pressure is the pressure within the arteries as the heart forces blood to circulate around your body.

How common is high blood pressure?

High blood pressure (or hypertension) is found right across the world and is particularly common in African–Caribbean and black American individuals. It is also, however, very common in the UK, with perhaps

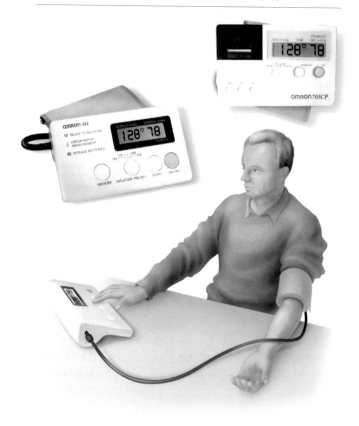

Electronic automatic blood pressure machines can be easy to use, but choose carefully to ensure accuracy (see recommendations on the website of the British Hypertension Society – see page 116).

25 per cent of the population over the age of 50 having high blood pressure readings.

The cause of high blood pressure is not known in most people. It does run in families and is seen in people with kidney disease. Unfortunately, in most cases high blood pressure gives rise to no symptoms, so it is sensible to have your blood pressure checked from time to time in case it is high and you don't know it.

Why is high blood pressure bad?

The high pressure in the arteries damages the lining and accelerates the development of atheroma (hardening of the arteries – see page 18). The heart also has to work harder to pump blood under high pressure, but it must do so without an adequate supply of oxygen. This increases the chances of developing angina or having a heart attack. High blood pressure also increases the risk of a stroke because of the damage that it causes to blood vessels in the brain. See the Family Doctor book *Understanding Blood Pressure*.

Diabetes

This is a common condition that affects roughly 3 in 100 people in the UK. It is caused by a deficiency of, or a resistance to, the hormone insulin, which is essential to control the movement of glucose into cells around the body via the bloodstream. Diabetes is strongly linked to being overweight and this is the reason why there is so much concern about the 'obesity epidemic' in children today.

Diabetes can affect people of any age, including children, and, the younger you are when you get diabetes, the more likely you are to need insulin injections to control it. Many people, however, get diabetes in middle or old age. When this happens, there are few symptoms and the condition can be controlled by diet and tablets. The aim of treatment is to keep the level of glucose in the blood as close as possible to normal. Nevertheless, despite treatment, diabetes can increase the risk of many circulatory disorders including CHD. For women this is particularly important because it seems to counteract the protective effect of female hormones and almost as many women as men with diabetes develop CHD.

Good control of diabetes, with diet, tablets or insulin, makes heart and circulatory problems less common. Poor control can often result in very abnormal blood fats, including cholesterol, and people with diabetes may need to take additional drugs to control this. See the Family Doctor book *Understanding Diabetes*.

KEY POINTS

- CHD is much more common in men than in women, and in old than in young people

- Important risk factors for CHD are smoking, raised blood cholesterol, high blood pressure and diabetes

- Stopping smoking and reducing cholesterol and blood pressure levels cut the risk of CHD

Recognising the symptoms

Although all people with coronary heart disease (CHD) have the same underlying problem, narrowing of the coronary arteries, they don't all get the same symptoms. Some develop angina, others may have a heart attack. A smaller proportion of people may develop heart failure without having any other warning symptoms. We don't really know why it affects people in different ways.

Chest pain

Not all chest pain is caused by CHD! No one would think that they had heart disease after falling and bruising their ribs, for example, and most of us have had indigestion which can sometimes give pain in the chest too.

You might think that it would be easy to distinguish chest pain caused by heart disease from that of any other cause, but in fact it can be difficult, even for the most experienced doctor.

How to recognise heart pain (angina)

The main features are:

- A dull pain that does not feel worse when you breathe in
- Usually in the middle of the chest but may spread to the left side, into both arms or up into the neck or jaw
- Could be described as: heavy, burning, vice like or like 'a weight on the chest'

Angina

Angina pectoris is simply Latin for pain in the chest. It is usually brought on by exercise, going away with rest. In angina, the pain comes from the muscle fibres in the heart, which don't have enough oxygen for the work that they are doing.

Angina usually lasts for about two or three minutes and generally no more than ten. It may come on only when you walk uphill, into a strong wind or when you're climbing stairs. It can sometimes come on after quite mild exertion, such as getting dressed if you have been resting a while. It is usually worse in the cold weather and if you exercise after a meal – taking the dog for a walk after breakfast, for example.

Unstable angina

In general, angina is fairly predictable, but, if the coronary artery narrows still further or a clot forms on its surface, then the disease can enter a new phase – unstable angina – and this can lead to a heart attack. You may suddenly find that you can walk only a short distance before developing pain, or you may develop

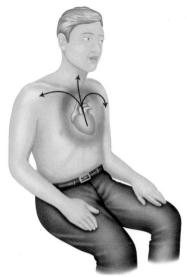

Pain from the heart is usually felt beneath the breast bone in the centre of the chest, but may spread into either arm (even to the finger tips) and to the jaw or back.

pain doing light work around the house or even going upstairs to bed. Sometimes you may be woken from sleep by an attack of angina. A change in the pattern of pain is an important development and should be reported to your doctor as soon as possible.

Heart attack

The pain is the same as angina, but, instead of easing off when you rest, it gets worse. People often say it is the worst pain they have ever felt in their lives. Someone who is having a heart attack may look grey and sweaty, and feel cold to the touch. They often feel sick and may vomit.

Some people who have heart attacks have never had any symptoms of heart disease – it just comes out

The stages of coronary heart disease

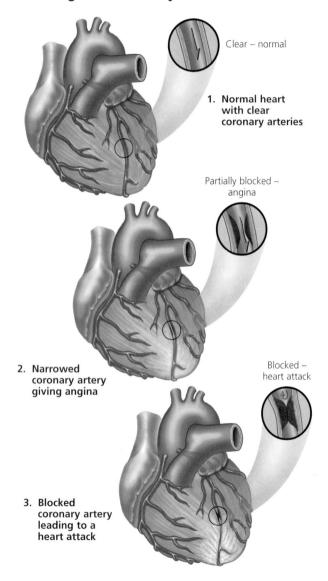

Clear – normal

1. **Normal heart with clear coronary arteries**

Partially blocked – angina

2. **Narrowed coronary artery giving angina**

Blocked – heart attack

3. **Blocked coronary artery leading to a heart attack**

of the blue. Most, however, will have had some pain off and on for weeks or months before as the blood vessels gradually narrowed, although they may not have realised that it was coming from the heart.

In about 20 per cent of cases, the symptoms of a heart attack may be mild and are often mistaken for indigestion. This is particularly true of elderly people and those with diabetes, perhaps because the pain fibres to the heart are not as sensitive as in young people.

Other causes of chest pain
We all experience pains in the chest from time to time as we do in other parts of our body. The most likely causes are the following.

Indigestion or 'heartburn'
The gullet (or oesophagus), which leads from the mouth to the stomach, lies just behind the heart and shares the same nerve supply. So it is not surprising that pain from the gullet – heartburn – may feel much like pain from the heart. Heartburn can occur at any time but is usually related to food, starting half an hour or so after meals or when the stomach is empty.

Heartburn can also occur at night when you lie flat because some of the acid from the stomach spills back into the gullet and irritates it. Eating more food or drinking milk or antacids eases heartburn, and hot fluids and alcohol make it worse.

Indigestion is not, however, brought on by exercise and if you feel a pain in your chest when you walk – even if it makes you belch – it is much more likely to be from your heart than from your stomach. See your doctor!

Pleurisy

Chest infections such as pneumonia can give rise to quite bad chest pain called pleurisy. The pain is usually sharp, only on one side of the chest, and is worse when you cough or take a deep breath. This is quite different from the dull constant pain from the heart which spreads right across the chest.

Muscle pain

Along the back and between the ribs there are muscles that play an important part in breathing and, like all muscles, they can be subject to rheumatic pain. This pain is usually confined to a fairly small area of the chest, either at the front or at the back. It is worse when sitting or lying in certain positions or when you turn round. It can last from a few hours to a few days and then may disappear before returning a few weeks later.

Less common causes of chest pain

There are other possible causes of chest pain, although they are less common.

Shingles

This viral infection can cause severe pain around the chest for two or three days before the tell-tale blistering rash appears in the painful area.

Viral infections

Some cold or flu-like viruses can affect the cartilage which attaches the ribs to the breastbone. When this happens, the chest will feel tender when you press it and the pain is quite different from angina.

Chest pain not related to the heart

Chest pain can be alarming and often causes people to believe that they are having a heart attack. However, there are many other, less serious, causes of chest pain.

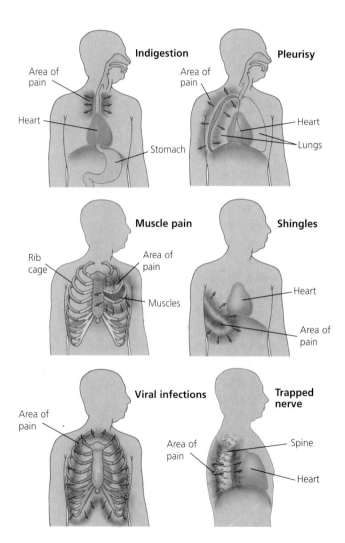

Indigestion
Area of pain
Heart
Stomach

Pleurisy
Area of pain
Heart
Lungs

Muscle pain
Rib cage
Area of pain
Muscles

Shingles
Heart
Area of pain

Viral infections
Area of pain

Trapped nerve
Spine
Area of pain
Heart

Trapped nerve

Sometimes, pressure on a nerve in the back or neck can cause pain that spreads down the arm or around the chest. This can be caused by damage to a disc or by arthritis in the spine. Another relatively common cause, particularly in older women, is collapse of a bone in the spine. This is usually the result of a condition called osteoporosis in which the bones become thin and fragile.

Palpitations

Palpitations – when the heart beats irregularly or misses a beat – are very common in healthy people. They are usually brought on by stress, smoking or drinking too much coffee and tea. A few people may also have an electrical 'short circuit' in the heart which gives rise to a very rapid heart beat, but this is uncommon.

People with CHD can also develop problems with heart rhythm but this is most likely in the first few days after a heart attack and your doctor will then give special drugs to try to control this. If palpitations are associated with faintness, breathlessness or chest pain, you should tell your doctor as soon as possible.

Breathlessness and swollen ankles

There are many possible reasons for breathlessness, of which the most common are chronic bronchitis, emphysema and asthma. Heart failure also causes breathlessness and can affect someone who has had a heart attack (see page 47). If the heart isn't pumping properly, fluid tends to build up in the tissues and lungs, and the result is breathlessness.

You may then find it difficult to lie flat in bed or wake up in the night with problems getting your breath. You may also develop a cough with a little frothy or blood-stained phlegm.

When fluid builds up elsewhere in the body, you may find that your ankles swell or that you get pain in the stomach because your liver and gut are swollen. When you are known to have a heart condition, increasing breathlessness or a cough that won't go away may be important. There are now effective drugs for treating heart failure and the sooner you seek help the better.

KEY POINTS

- When the heart muscle is short of oxygen, the result is chest pain – angina

- Severe chest pain is a heart attack until proved otherwise

- Angina pain usually comes on when you exercise or are under stress

- Indigestion is not usually brought on by exercise; if in doubt seek advice

Tests for CHD

Identifying the cause of chest pains

There are many possible causes of chest pain and the most important clue lies in the nature of the pain itself and when it comes on (see pages 45–53). Doctors are usually able to distinguish between the different types of pain in the chest. It may be clear, simply from what you tell the doctor, that the pain is coming from your heart or from some other cause.

The pain from a heart attack or from angina is often unmistakable. However, there are other times when the diagnosis is less clear cut and the doctor then has to make a decision based upon how likely it is that you might have coronary heart disease (CHD). In a young woman, chest pain is much more likely to be indigestion than angina whereas, in a middle-aged man who smokes and has high blood pressure, it is more likely to be angina than indigestion.

Experience counts, but unfortunately no doctor is infallible, and many doctors have not even been able to diagnose their own heart attack! But, because CHD is so common in the UK, most doctors will arrange further tests if there is any doubt about the diagnosis.

Heart tracing
Resting ECG

The most common test for heart conditions is the electrocardiograph or ECG for short (in America it is called the EKG). It is a simple, painless test that takes about 10 minutes and can be done by your GP or practice nurse.

Every time the heart beats, it causes natural electrical changes that can be picked up by electrodes placed at various points around the body. These electrodes, covered in a sticky gel to ensure good contact, are usually put on the ankles, wrists and across the chest.

The tracing records the heart rate and rhythm and whether the muscle is conducting electricity normally. Damaged muscle or muscle that is short of oxygen will result in a different appearance.

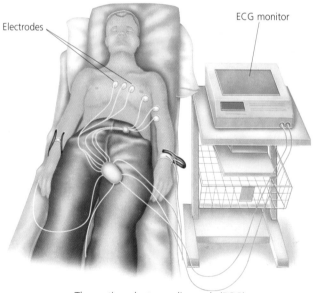

Electrodes

ECG monitor

The resting electrocardiograph (ECG).

The ECG tracing gives the doctor a lot of information about the heart, but, like most tests, the ECG is not infallible. If you have angina, your heart trace may still be normal if it is recorded at rest when free of pain. In this case, you may need an exercise ECG.

Exercise ECG

Any form of exercise can be used to provoke angina. In the UK, we generally use a treadmill test, but in Europe they often use a bicycle. ECG electrodes are attached just as for the resting ECG, but the wires are attached carefully to the chest so that they don't come loose while you are walking. The treadmill usually starts at a slow pace on the flat and then increases every two or three

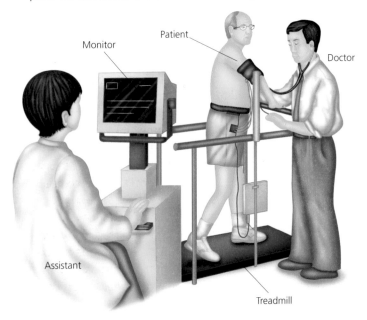

Monitor

Patient

Doctor

Assistant

Treadmill

Exercise ECG: as you walk your heart rate and electrical activity are measured via electrodes.

minutes to a faster speed on an increasing slope so that you are effectively walking uphill. The test is stopped if you develop pain, if there are major ECG changes or, of course, if you become tired or too breathless.

The useful thing about the exercise ECG is that it gives two bits of information to the doctor. The first is that, if the test produces pain and ECG changes, it confirms the diagnosis of angina. The second and just as important is that, if you manage to walk a fair distance before the pain comes on, it tells the doctor that the angina is mild and further tests may not be necessary.

The test is done as a hospital outpatient and takes about 40 minutes.

Radioactive isotope tests

These tests make use of chemicals, or isotopes, which give out very small amounts of radioactivity that can be picked up by a special camera. Different tissues around the body take up different isotopes. For the heart various isotopes are used, the most common being thallium and technetium. Both these are taken up by heart muscle with a normal blood supply but would not be taken up by muscle that has a poor blood supply. So where there is a narrowing or blockage of a coronary artery, that area of heart muscle will not show up.

Isotopes are radioactive, but the amount of radioactivity given in these tests is small and equivalent to most standard X-ray procedures. The isotope breaks down quickly in the body and some of it is passed in the urine, but it does not pose any danger to you or anybody else.

The isotope scan is carried out in two stages, once when the heart is stressed and once again when it is at

Radioactive isotope tests

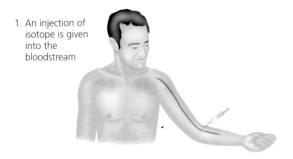

1. An injection of isotope is given into the bloodstream

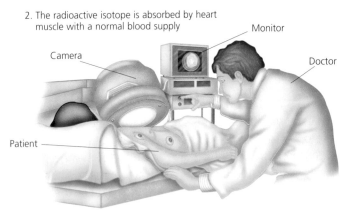

2. The radioactive isotope is absorbed by heart muscle with a normal blood supply

Monitor

Camera

Doctor

Patient

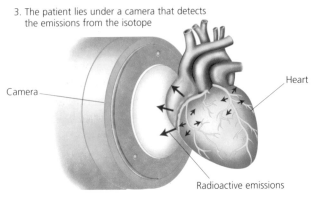

3. The patient lies under a camera that detects the emissions from the isotope

Heart

Camera

Radioactive emissions

rest, and the two images are compared. The stress pictures are usually taken after a treadmill test but, for those who can't exercise, the heart can be stimulated by drugs, such as adenosine, dipyridamole and dobutamine. At the end of the exercise test or after receiving the drug, an injection of isotope is given and you then lie under the camera for 10 or 15 minutes while the pictures are taken.

Sometimes, the isotope scan is better at picking up abnormalities than the exercise ECG, and it is useful after bypass surgery when the arterial supply to the heart can become quite complicated. It is also the only way to study the heart in people who can't manage the treadmill or bicycle, for example, because of arthritis or bad lung disease.

Stress echocardiography

This is a technique that is similar in principle to the isotope test, except that radioactivity is not involved. Echocardiography is the name given to the scanner which uses sound beams to take pictures of the heart and is just the same as the ultrasound scanner used to see the baby in a mother's uterus.

With this type of scanner, it is possible to see the heart muscle contracting and to pick out any parts that are contracting poorly because the blood supply has been cut off. As in the isotope study, the heart can be stimulated either by exercise or by the injection of drugs and the heart is scanned before, during and after the stress. The pictures are then analysed in detail and can give good information as to which arteries may be blocked and how badly.

Echocardiography

An instrument called a transducer, which produces a beam of sound, is held against the chest. A picture of the heart is created by the reflected sound beams.

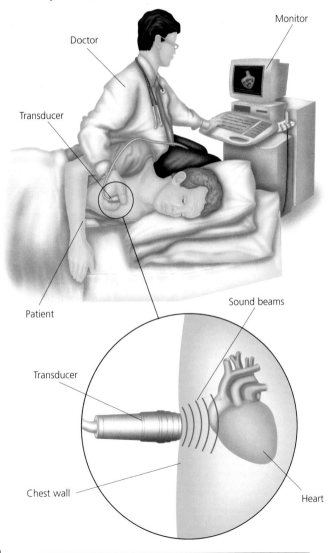

Doctor

Monitor

Transducer

Patient

Sound beams

Transducer

Chest wall

Heart

Coronary angiography

The most direct way of finding out what is wrong with the heart in CHD is to undertake special X-rays of the coronary arteries, called angiograms. These X-rays are taken after dye that can be seen on an X-ray is injected directly into the coronary arteries. As the heart is moving all the time, the X-rays have to be taken on video, so it requires expensive equipment that at one time was available only in a few large teaching hospitals. With modern technology, these facilities are more widely available and most district hospitals can now undertake angiography.

In order to take a picture of these small arteries, the dye needs to be injected directly into them. To do this, a fine tube (two to three millimetres in diameter) called a catheter has to be passed to the heart, usually from an artery in the groin, or sometimes from an artery in the wrist. A little local anaesthetic is injected under the skin to numb it. The catheter is then passed up along the artery towards the heart. You will not be aware of this happening, although when the tube reaches the heart you may have a few palpitations. This is quite normal.

Once the catheter is in the coronary artery, dye is injected and pictures taken from various angles. While this is being done, you will be asked to hold your breath for perhaps five or ten seconds. The dye may cause a little flushing which passes off quickly.

Coronary angiography is a safe and routine procedure. Serious complications are rare – less than one in 1,000. The most important risk, which fortunately is very uncommon, is that the angiogram can provoke a heart attack or stroke. If this should happen, emergency surgery may be needed. Less

Coronary angiography

A catheter is passed from an artery in the groin to the heart.
A dye is injected into the coronary arteries. The dye is revealed
by an X-ray camera that is able to produce moving images.

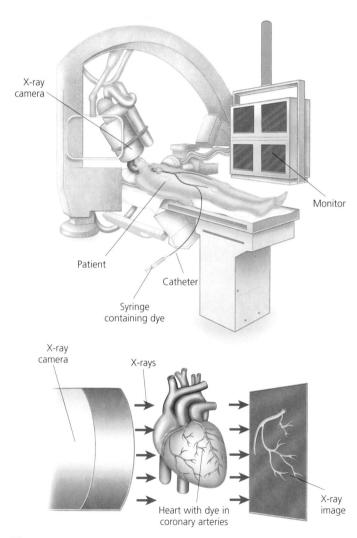

X-ray
camera

Monitor

Patient

Catheter

Syringe
containing dye

X-ray
camera

X-rays

Heart with dye in
coronary arteries

X-ray
image

serious complications are an allergy to the dye or damage to the artery at the puncture site.

Coronary angiography is often done as a day-case procedure and takes 30 to 60 minutes. You probably won't have to stay in hospital overnight but you will need to lie down for three or four hours afterwards to reduce the risk of any bleeding from the groin or wrist. The area used for the test will often be bruised and may be a little tender for a few days.

Although coronary angiography is the best way of looking at the coronary arteries, it is not necessary for everyone with angina or CHD. Most doctors will use it only where they think that it is likely that you might benefit from heart surgery or angioplasty (see pages 73–5).

KEY POINTS

- The most common test for heart disease is the ECG, but it is not infallible

- If the resting ECG is normal, a treadmill exercise test is a good way to show angina and see how serious it is

- For anyone who can't exercise, radioisotope testing or echocardiography may be used instead

- Coronary angiography is the best way of identifying which arteries are affected, but is not needed by everyone with CHD

Treating angina

Angina is pain in the chest caused by too little oxygen reaching the heart muscle. It usually comes on after exercise and disappears when you have rested for a few minutes. Unstable angina is when the condition gets rapidly worse so that eventually you are in pain even when resting. It may be a warning of an impending heart attack.

The doctor's aim when treating angina is to relieve the pain itself and to increase the amount of exercise that you can do before pain starts. Treatment may be with drugs (medical treatment), angioplasty or surgery.

Medical treatments

Usually drug treatment will be tried first. Drugs work by reducing the amount of oxygen needed by the heart muscle or increasing the blood flow to the heart, or both.

There are basically three types of drugs used in patients with angina:

- A drug for the pain itself such as glyceryl trinitrate (GTN)

- A drug such as a statin to lower cholesterol

- A drug to prevent clots forming, usually aspirin.

Whatever treatment your doctor starts you on, it is important that you work together as a partnership. You must take your medication as prescribed – in most cases, this is likely to be once or twice a day. If there are any side effects you should report them promptly.

You should also make any necessary adjustments to your lifestyle. This might mean giving up smoking, losing weight and taking more exercise. You will find more about this in the chapter beginning on page 98.

Nitrates

Nitrates are the most common drugs to relieve the pain of angina and have been used in various forms for more than 100 years. Glyceryl trinitrate (or GTN for short) is absorbed very quickly through the lining of the mouth and is taken either as a small tablet under the tongue or as a spray. It dilates, or opens up, the coronary arteries and so improves the blood flow to the heart muscle in areas where the coronary arteries are narrowed.

Nitrates also dilate the arteries and veins throughout the body and this can lead to side effects, particularly dizziness and headache. If you do feel dizzy after using GTN sit or lie down for a few minutes and the effect will usually pass off. The headache after using GTN is caused by the blood vessels to the brain dilating. It usually comes on within a minute or two of taking the nitrate and disappears quickly if you spit the tablet out.

People often find that the pain from angina starts to ease as the headache comes on. The effect of nitrates is so predictable in CHD that doctors often use this to tell

The effect of nitrates on the heart

In cases of angina, when the blood vessels supplying the heart are constricted, nitrates can be taken to dilate the blood vessels and increase the flow of blood to the heart. As more oxygen becomes available, the strain on the heart is reduced.

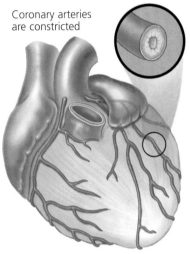

Coronary arteries are constricted

Heart muscle is starved of oxygen

During an angina attack

Nitrates dilate the coronary arteries

Normal blood supply returns to the heart muscle

Afer taking nitrates

whether your chest pain is really angina. This is a fairly reliable test but pain from the gullet (oesophagus) can sometimes be eased by GTN which can be confusing.

Anyone who has angina should always keep their GTN tablets or spray with them wherever they are in case they get an unexpected attack of chest pain. However, if you have opened a bottle of tablets but not used any for a while, do keep an eye on the expiry date – GTN tablets will not work once the bottle has been open for more than six weeks.

As we have seen, GTN works very quickly indeed, so if the pain has not settled within five minutes of taking the medicine, it may be developing into something more serious. Your doctor will probably advise you to wait for five minutes and if there has been no improvement to take another dose.

IF THE CHEST PAIN IS STILL NO BETTER 10 MINUTES AFTER A SECOND DOSE OF GTN, YOU SHOULD SEEK IMMEDIATE MEDICAL HELP.

Nitrates can be swallowed as a tablet but are not absorbed all that well from the stomach, which is why other, more effective ways of taking them have been developed. Special formulations include a longer-acting tablet that can be left between the gums and the cheek for several hours (called buccal nitrate). There is even a skin patch containing GTN. This is a transparent plaster containing the drug that is absorbed slowly through the skin. It is left on for 18 hours and is usually removed at night. Your doctor may try several different nitrates to find out which suits you best.

Beta blockers

Beta blockers are a group of drugs that were discovered in the UK over 30 years ago and were a major advance in the treatment of angina. They were called beta blockers because they block the effects of adrenaline (epinephrine) on so-called beta-receptors in the heart, lungs and blood vessels. Their effect is to slow down the heart beat and reduce the blood pressure, particularly during exercise, so enabling the heart to undertake more work before angina comes on. People with angina usually find that they can walk further than they could before, and have to use their GTN less often. Sometimes, people find that their angina disappears altogether, though it would probably come on if they exercised hard enough.

Unfortunately, beta blockers do not suit everybody. They cannot be given to people with bronchitis or asthma as they can make breathing worse. Other possible side effects include cold hands and feet, aching in the leg muscles when walking, tiredness and, occasionally, impotence. There are, however, more than a dozen different beta blockers available at present and often people find that one suits them better than another.

Calcium channel blockers

Calcium channel blockers slow down the rate at which calcium can enter body cells, particularly in the heart muscle and blood vessel walls. This group of drugs acts rather like nitrates by dilating the coronary arteries and improving the blood flow to the heart muscle. Like beta blockers they increase the amount of exercise that you can manage before getting angina although they do not slow the heart rate. As they act in a different way, they can be used with beta blockers or nitrates.

How nitrates can be taken

Nitrates are available in a variety of formulations.

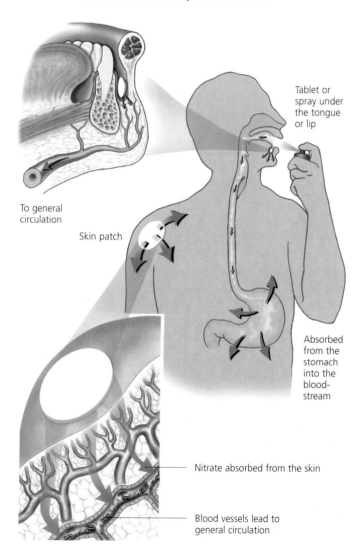

Tablet or spray under the tongue or lip

To general circulation

Skin patch

Absorbed from the stomach into the blood-stream

Nitrate absorbed from the skin

Blood vessels lead to general circulation

The most common side effects, as with nitrates, are headaches and dizziness. They can also cause swelling of the ankles and constipation.

Nicorandil

Nicorandil is one of the newer drugs and acts a bit like nitrates and calcium channel blockers to dilate the coronary arteries. It does so, however, by a different mechanism and may work when nitrates don't. In some patients it reduces the risk of heart attacks.

Aspirin

Aspirin should be taken by everyone with angina, provided that it does not upset them. It works by 'thinning' the blood so that it clots less easily. The danger for someone with angina is that a clot will form in any narrowed coronary artery and lead to a heart attack. By reducing the risk of clots forming, aspirin reduces the risk of a heart attack.

The amount of aspirin needed to do this is only 75 milligrams a day – a quarter of an ordinary aspirin tablet. At these low doses side effects are rare but there are some people who are allergic to aspirin (especially those with asthma) or who find that it gives them indigestion.

Clopidogrel

Clopidogrel acts in a similar manner to aspirin to thin the blood, but it does not cause as much indigestion. New research also shows that it is very useful in unstable angina when used in combination with aspirin. So, if you have recently been in hospital with angina, you may well come out taking both. It is also used in most patients who have had an angioplasty (see page 73).

Other drugs

Other drugs are being developed all the time for the treatment of angina and your doctor may wish to use one of these in your case, either because others have not worked or because they have had side effects.

In some situations your doctor may also give you additional drugs to control your blood pressure more effectively. A common choice would be the angiotensin-converting enzyme inhibitors (ACE inhibitors for short) and there is some evidence that these drugs help to prevent any deterioration in your heart condition. (See page 88 for more details of these drugs.)

Surgical treatments

By no means everyone with angina will need an operation but, where the symptoms are becoming difficult to control with drugs, the results of surgery can be dramatic. An individual who has had angina for years, for example, can walk without difficulty again and some, such as Sir Ranulph Fiennes, have even completed several marathons! There are now many procedures that can be used to improve blood flow, either by bypassing arteries (coronary artery bypass surgery or CABG) or by stretching them (coronary angioplasty or PCI).

Although both CABG and PCI work well, they are not really a 'cure' in the sense that they do not get rid of the basic problem which is the 'furring' up of the coronary arteries.

You still need to take all the steps necessary to prevent the arteries from deteriorating, either by changes in lifestyle such as stopping smoking, or with drugs such as those to lower cholesterol.

Angioplasty
What does it involve?
Angioplasty was first used about 25 years ago and involves stretching narrowed areas of blood vessels to improve blood flow. This is much quicker and easier than CABG but may be less reliable in the long term.

In principle, angioplasty is a technique whereby a long, thin balloon is passed across the narrowed region of a blood vessel, over a very fine guidewire. The balloon is then inflated at high pressure and stretches the artery, often splitting the fatty deposits in its wall. When the balloon is deflated and removed, the artery remains open.

How effective is angioplasty?
The problem with coronary angioplasty is that, in about one in four people, the narrowing may come back within a few weeks or months. Either the artery is not stretched far enough in the first place or inflammation sets in. This has, however, been largely prevented by the use of coronary stents which are now used routinely in most patients.

A stent is a fine wire mesh that is stretched over the balloon and, as the balloon is blown up, it stretches with the artery and remains there to hold it open once the balloon has been removed. Newer, specially coated stents have reduced the risks of recurrence substantially, making angioplasty an effective long-term treatment for patients with angina.

Having an angioplasty
The operation is usually done on an overnight basis – you go in in the morning and come home the next

Coronary angioplasty and stent placement

Angioplasty involves stretching the affected artery by inserting a balloon along a guide wire and then inflating it at the site of the blockage.

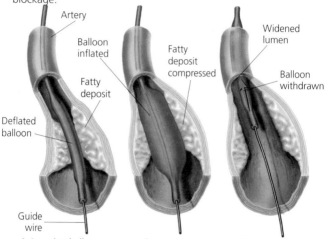

Artery

Balloon inflated

Fatty deposit

Deflated balloon

Guide wire

1. Inserting balloon

Fatty deposit compressed

2. Inflating balloon

Widened lumen

Balloon withdrawn

3. Withdrawing balloon

Sometimes a fine wire mesh stent is used to hold the artery open and prevent any recurrence.

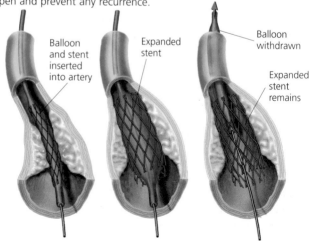

Balloon and stent inserted into artery

1. Stent and deflated balloon in place

Expanded stent

2. Balloon inflated, stretches stent

Balloon withdrawn

Expanded stent remains

3. Deflated balloon removed. Stent left in artery

day. From your point of view, the procedure is exactly the same as having coronary angiography (see page 61):

- A deflated balloon is passed with a fine wire into narrowed areas of the blood vessels and inflated.

- It is then removed – and you won't have felt any of this happening. Sometimes you may experience some chest pain during the procedure and there is a very small chance that angioplasty may cause a sudden blockage, necessitating an emergency CABG. Usually, however, you'll be back to normal after a week.

- Angioplasty can be repeated later, more than once if necessary.

Who is suitable for angioplasty?

Unfortunately, angioplasty is not suitable for everybody. It is best for people with one or two areas of narrowing in large arteries, and is really no good for those who have small diameter vessels or narrowing in all three coronary arteries. In these circumstances bypass surgery may be a better long-term solution.

Bypass surgery
What does it involve?

Bypass surgery has been one of the major advances in the treatment of angina. The name comes from the type of operation that 'bypasses' the blockages in the coronary arteries using replacement blood vessels taken from the chest wall or the legs.

When the operation was first performed surgeons used veins removed from the leg. These were cut into lengths of 4 to 5 inches (10 to 13 centimetres) and

Coronary bypass surgery

A section of vein is taken from the leg and grafted to the aorta and coronary artery.

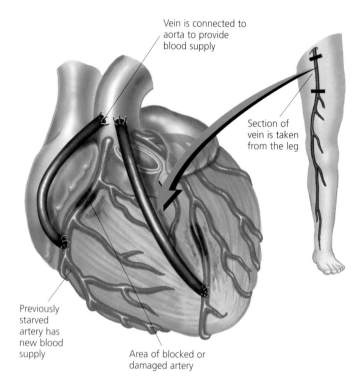

Vein is connected to aorta to provide blood supply

Section of vein is taken from the leg

Previously starved artery has new blood supply

Area of blocked or damaged artery

sewn between the blocked coronary arteries and the aorta (the main artery leading from the heart to the rest of the body).

In the last 10 years techniques have changed and, whenever possible, most surgeons now use small arteries rather than vein grafts. The long-term results of this technique appear to be better than with veins, which were never made to withstand the pressures normally present in the coronary arteries.

Coronary bypass surgery

Showing one graft from the internal mammary artery.

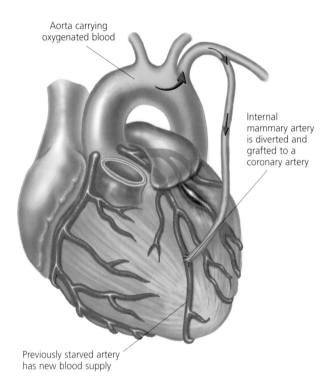

Aorta carrying oxygenated blood

Internal mammary artery is diverted and grafted to a coronary artery

Previously starved artery has new blood supply

The two most commonly used arteries are the internal mammary arteries, which run down behind the breast bone. They can be attached to either the left or right coronary artery. More recently surgeons have also used arteries from the arm. All of these are likely to last longer than the vein grafts.

What are the risks of surgery?

Major heart surgery is not without risks and would not

be recommended for everyone with angina, particularly if the symptoms were mild. There are, however, some people with mild angina who need bypass surgery because they have a high risk of a heart attack. This is usually because angiography has shown that all three coronary arteries are affected.

A few people still have angina after CABG because it may not be possible to bypass all the blockages. Bypassing all the main arteries will reduce the risk of further heart attacks but some of the arteries may be too small to operate on, so mild angina may still occur, although it can usually be controlled with drugs.

Unfortunately the new blood vessels may not last for ever and if they do narrow or block a second operation may be needed. A second bypass can be more risky than the first, but using the new technique with mammary arteries, the long-term results can be just as good or better.

Having a CABG

- Usually, you will be admitted to hospital for one or two days before your operation for final tests and assessment.

- On the day itself, you will go to sleep in the anaesthetic room and wake up in the ITU (intensive therapy unit), probably still on a ventilator which is doing your breathing for you.

- You often have a lot of drips, drains and monitors for the first 24 hours or so, but after that most should be removed and you will go back to the ward.

- After five to ten days, you'll be able to go home and, around six to eight weeks later, you should be back to most of your normal activities. In other words, you can drive, go back to work provided that it doesn't involve heavy manual labour and resume your sex life. For a fuller discussion of heart surgery see the Family Doctor Book *Understanding Heart Surgery.*

KEY POINTS

- Glyceryl trinitrate (GTN) taken as a tablet or spray under the tongue eases the pain of angina quickly, and should be carried at all times

- Nitrates, beta blockers and calcium channel blockers are very effective alone, and in combination, in controlling angina

- Angioplasty (PCI) is a technique where the narrowed artery is stretched by a high-pressure balloon, and is very effective in certain situations, particularly with a stent

- Coronary bypass surgery (CABG) is very effective in relieving angina and is particularly suitable for advanced disease

Treating a heart attack

Emergency assistance

If you have severe pain in the chest, and feel cold, sweaty and nauseated, you are probably having a heart attack. This happens when a coronary artery becomes blocked, usually in an already narrowed vessel. The ambulance staff, paramedics or GP or a combination of all three may come to attend to you but their aims are the same: to stabilise your heart and reduce the amount of damage done to the muscle if at all possible.

When medical help arrives, you will be given oxygen via a facemask and have a plastic cannula (tube) inserted into a vein in your arm so that any drugs needed can go straight into your bloodstream. You will have ECG leads attached to your chest to monitor your heart rhythm and may be given morphine for the pain as well as something to stop the sickness.

Dissolving the clot

In the early stages, the most important treatment is to dissolve the clot and, in some cases, this may be

Treatment priorities

The priorities of the medical care team in treating a heart attack patient are to:

- Relieve pain and other symptoms, such as nausea
- Treat any serious cardiac irregularities promptly, with a defibrillator if necessary
- Restore blood supply to the affected heart muscle by dissolving the clot in the coronary artery
- Treat complications of the heart attack such as irregular heartbeat or heart failure

started before you reach hospital. Although it may sound odd, chewing an aspirin tablet is a good way to start. It is absorbed through the lining of the mouth and starts to thin the blood immediately.

In addition to aspirin, we have many new drugs available. The last 15 years have seen a dramatic change in the way that we treat heart attacks because we now have powerful drugs that dissolve the clot that is at the root of the problem. These drugs are called thrombolytics (often referred to as 'clot busters') and are given by injection. The most common in this country is streptokinase or tPa (tissue plasminogen activator).

The essential point about thrombolytics is that they work best if given within the first six hours after a heart attack. This is because, after this, the heart may be too badly damaged to recover, even if the artery is unblocked again. For that reason thrombolytics are now given at home by paramedics in some areas to reduce the delay to a minimum.

The effect of 'clot-buster' drugs

In the early stages of a heart attack powerful drugs can be used to dissolve the clot that is the cause of the problem.

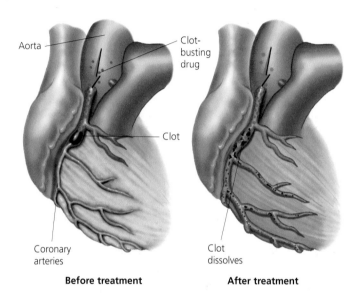

Aorta

Clot-busting drug

Clot

Coronary arteries

Clot dissolves

Before treatment

After treatment

The use of these powerful drugs is not without some risk but large trials involving tens of thousands of patients with heart attacks have shown that the benefits greatly outweigh the risks.

As thrombolytics dissolve blood clots they do make people more liable to bleed. In some individuals, this may pose too great a risk – for instance, if someone has recently had a major operation, a stroke or a bleeding stomach ulcer. In these situations, it may be possible to undertake immediate angioplasty, if you are in a hospital where this is carried out (see page 73).

Streptokinase card

If you are given streptokinase, you will be given a card to show that you have had it and when. This is because most people develop resistance to streptokinase after five days or so and this resistance lasts for a year or more.

So if you need thrombolytic drugs within this period you will be given the alternative, tPa.

IT IS VERY IMPORTANT THAT YOU CARRY THIS CARD WITH YOU AT ALL TIMES IN CASE YOU ARE TAKEN INTO HOSPITAL AGAIN.

Regulating the heart beat

In the early stages after a heart attack, the damaged heart muscle can become very irritable and produce irregular heart rhythms, some of which can cause the heart to stop completely. Sadly this is why some people die suddenly at home after developing chest pain before any help has arrived. These irregularities of heart rhythm – cardiac arrhythmias – can be treated very successfully by passing a brief electric shock through the heart using a gadget called a defibrillator – something that you may well have seen on a film or on TV.

People who need this treatment have always lost consciousness, so no anaesthetic is necessary. Unfortunately, the procedure works only if the shock can be given within a few minutes of the heart stopping, which is why the 999 ambulance and paramedic services are so vital. IF YOU KNOW WHAT TO DO, YOU MAY ALSO BE ABLE TO GIVE VITAL HELP (SEE PAGES 112–13).

In hospital, people who have had a heart attack are usually treated in a special ward (the cardiac care unit

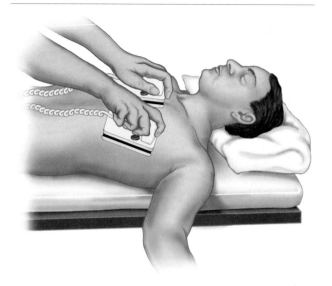

A defibrillator is sometimes used to make the heart start beating
normally. It works by administering an electrical shock to the
region of the heart via two metal plates that are placed on the
patient's chest.

or CCU) where the heart rhythms can be monitored
closely for the first 24 or 48 hours – the danger period. If
irregular rhythms develop they can usually be controlled
with drug treatment and won't become severe enough
to need a shock. After this the risk of rhythm problems
becomes much less and drugs such as beta blockers
are used to prevent them happening again.

Recovering in hospital

The worst period after a heart attack is the first day or
two; during this time, you will usually be monitored closely.
After that most people have no more pain and get up
and about fairly quickly. After a straightforward heart
attack, you may be able to go home after five days,

but some people, particularly elderly people, may need to stay in hospital longer.

In the first week, although there is no more pain, you may feel tired and have a slight temperature, but this feeling usually settles as the healing process begins. The damaged area of heart muscle is repaired and a scar forms just like on any other part of the body after an injury. This scarring is more or less complete four to six weeks after the heart attack.

If this is the first time that you have been in hospital or had anything seriously wrong, it may take some time to come to terms with what has happened, especially if you have financial and family commitments to worry about too. Nursing and medical staff are well aware of these worries and you should feel free to talk about them. It is time too to think about your lifestyle and what you can do to prevent another heart attack (see the chapter starting on page 98).

Going home

After all the attention in hospital, it often feels strange to be going back home. You will naturally be worried about what you can and can't do, and your spouse or partner may be even more worried than you! In fact it is usually quite safe to do most things around the house, but any heavy physical activity should be avoided in the first few weeks. Remember that this includes some housework such as vacuum cleaning, which uses more energy than you might think.

It is very important in these early stages that your family and friends try not to be too overprotective towards you. For them and for you, every little twinge of pain may seem larger than life. Most people after a heart attack become much more aware of aches and pains that they would previously have ignored. Indeed it has been reported that 90 per cent of people experience some form of non-cardiac pain in the first few weeks after a heart attack.

However, about one in three people get angina, which may feel similar to a heart attack. It will usually come on with effort, and ease when you rest. If so, you should take the GTN that you will have been given in hospital. If the pain persists after using GTN, take another, and if it lasts more than 20 minutes you should get immediate medical advice. There may be a helpline to the cardiac unit in your area and it is worth asking about this before you leave hospital.

Taking medicines when you go home

During the first week in hospital you will be given a number of different drugs, some to treat any complications and others to reduce the risk of further problems over the next weeks and months.

There is now a wide variety of drugs that may be given to people who have had a heart attack, and your doctor will decide which ones will do you the most good. Don't be surprised if you know someone who has been given different treatment as drugs must be tailored to suit the needs of each individual.

Aspirin

This is the most commonly prescribed drug, but some people can't take it, usually because they have stomach problems. Its main purpose is to reduce the stickiness of platelets – the cells in the blood that are involved in clotting. The new drug clopidrogel may now be an alternative.

Drugs that your doctor may prescribe

Class of drug	Generic name*	Administration
Anti-platelet drugs	Aspirin	Tablets
	Clopidogrel	Tablets
Nitrates	Glyceryl trinitrate (GTN)	Under the tongue, in the cheek, tablets, skin patches, ointment or spray
	Isosorbide dinitrate	Tablets, capsules or under the tongue
	Isosorbide mononitrate	Tablets or capsules
	Pentaerythritol tetranitrate	Tablets
Beta blockers	Acebutolol	Tablets or capsules
	Atenolol	Tablets or syrup
	Bisoprolol	Tablets
	Carvedilol	Tablets
	Metoprolol	Tablets
	Propranolol	Tablets or capsules
Calcium antagonists	Amlodipine	Tablets
	Diltiazem	Tablets or capsules
	Nicardipine	Capsules
	Nifedipine	Tablets or capsules
	Verapamil	Tablets or capsules
Potassium channel activators	Nicorandil	Tablets
ACE inhibitors	Captopril	Tablets
	Cilazapril	Tablets
	Enalapril	Tablets
	Fosinopril	Tablets
	Lisinopril	Tablets
	Perindopril	Tablets
	Quinapril	Tablets
	Ramipril	Capsules
	Trandolapril	Capsules
Statins	Atorvastatin	Tablets
	Fluvastatin	Capsules
	Pravastatin	Tablets
	Rosuvastatin	Tablets
	Simvastatin	Tablets

*Pharmaceutical companies all give their products 'proprietary/trade' names here; you will be able to find this on the package of your medication.

Drugs that your doctor may prescribe (contd)

Purpose	Possible side effects
Thin blood	Gastric upset
Relieve angina	Flushing, headache
Slow heart rate, protect against heart attack	Tiredness, lethargy, cold hands, nightmares
Relieve angina	Flushing, headache, ankle swelling, constipation
Relieve angina	Headache, dizziness, vomiting
Protect against heart failure	Persistent dry cough, dizziness
Reduce cholesterol	Headache, indigestion, occasionally muscle inflammation

as well their actual 'generic/scientific' name. Only the generic name is listed

Beta blockers

These are drugs that block the effect of adrenaline on receptors in the heart and blood vessels, thus reducing the risk of another heart attack and cutting the death rate. Many physicians prescribe them routinely after a heart attack but some people can't take them, for example, if they have asthma or bronchitis.

ACE inhibitors

These drugs have been a major advance in the treatment of heart problems. ACE – angiotensin-converting enzyme – increases the amount of angiotensin in the circulation. Angiotensin makes the blood vessels constrict and causes the body to retain more salt and water than normal. ACE inhibitors, by reducing the angiotensin levels, have cut the number of people developing heart attack and heart failure.

Statins

These are potent new drugs that lower cholesterol. They act by reducing the amount of cholesterol that is made in the liver and help to prevent arteries furring up any further (see page 18).

GTN

This is one of the most important drugs that you will be taking home, either as a spray or in tablet form. This is to use with any further pain in the chest after you leave hospital.

You should make sure that you know how and when to take GTN before you leave the hospital, and perhaps even try it so that you know what to expect. The doctors, nurses or pharmacist will answer your questions.

KEY POINTS

After a heart attack:

■ Prompt treatment is vital; ring 999 rather than your GP

■ Close monitoring is required in the first few days, usually in a cardiac care unit (CCU)

■ Most people can expect to recover fully in six to eight weeks

■ Drugs are important to prevent a recurrence

Getting over a heart attack

Rehabilitation

At one time doctors would have insisted that you stay in bed for six to eight weeks after a heart attack in the mistaken belief that this would allow the heart to heal better. It was not surprising that after such a long period in bed people felt worse than they did before they had the attack!

Things are very different now. Once the pain and general weakness have gone – usually a matter of a few days – the emphasis is on returning to normal over the next six to eight weeks.

Most hospitals now have a cardiac rehabilitation service – 'rehab' for short. The aims of cardiac rehabilitation are:

- Education: understanding the cause of the problem and how you are going to get better.

- Exercise: a graded exercise programme so that you can return to your normal activities.

- Prevention: how to avoid having a further heart attack.

The rehab programme usually begins in hospital when a nurse will visit you and try to answer some of the questions that must be troubling you and your family. You should be given some guidance about what sort of things you can and can't do when you leave hospital.

The exercise programme usually starts two to four weeks later and is supervised by a physiotherapist in the hospital gym. There will probably be a group of 10 to 15 other people going through the programme and it is a good time to talk together and share experiences. It is often very reassuring to see someone exercising quite energetically as they come to the end of the programme when you are just starting and are worried about doing any exercise at all.

For many middle-aged people, this may be the first regular exercise that they have done for years and so it will seem strange at first. However, most people find that the exercise becomes easier and easier as the weeks go by and are likely to feel fitter at the end of the programme than they have done for years.

Rehabilitation sessions usually last one to two hours and take place about twice a week for six to eight weeks. As well as the exercise itself there is usually time to have some discussion about the cause of heart attacks and what can be done to prevent them.

There may also be visits to a pharmacist, a dietitian and a cardiologist to answer any questions that you or your partner may have about your condition.

Special problems
Driving
You should not drive your car for one month after a heart attack. You do not need to notify the DVLA but

you should tell your insurance company. There are special regulations for people who drive for a living, such as bus drivers and lorry drivers, and you should discuss these with your doctor. In some towns these regulations also apply to taxi drivers as well.

Sexual activity

After a heart attack people worry about having sex. At first you don't usually feel like it but it is certainly reasonable to start sexual relations again three to four weeks after a heart attack if you want to. You should avoid being too vigorous until you feel fully recovered, which will normally be by about six to eight weeks. Some of the drugs that you may be taking can reduce sex drive and if you feel that this is the case you should have a word with your doctor.

Work

After a heart attack most people can go back to work after two or three months. For those with a physically undemanding job that does not involve much exercise eight weeks off work may be enough. For heavy manual workers longer may be necessary and special exercises are included in the exercise programme to build up their strength again. (Interestingly one of the first and most successful exercise programmes in Britain was in Barnsley to help miners get back to work.)

Holidays

For the first two or three months after a heart attack it is probably safest not to go abroad. Later you can probably travel where you like provided that you have made a full recovery. If in doubt, discuss your plans with your doctor. You should always make sure that you are fully insured and that the policy does not exclude a heart condition! If you are on medication, make sure that you have enough to last while you're away, and keep them in your hand luggage.

Anxiety and depression

In the first few weeks after a heart attack, there are so many things going on and so much to think about that depression may not be obvious. However, once things start to get back to normal, you may have more time to worry about the future, and this is when problems can occur.

The most common reaction is a short temper, even in people who have been quite placid, and partners often complain that they get their 'head bitten off' for the slightest thing. These problems usually settle down if and when the person returns to work, and life starts getting back to normal, but some people continue to have a 'short fuse' for much longer.

Everyone worries after a heart attack and, despite all the positive advice from doctors, nurses and relatives, some people go on worrying. There is bound to be some concern about having another heart attack, and all that it entails. It's natural to be worried about yourself and your family, even if it's difficult to put into words exactly why. A heart attack can be a real blow to your self-confidence, especially if you have never had any serious health problems before, and it's relatively easy to become depressed.

Recognising depression

Depression is just as much a real illness as heart disease, and also just as treatable. You may be depressed if you have several of the following symptoms:

- sadness or tearfulness
- loss of enjoyment or interest in work and hobbies
- low self-esteem
- preoccupation with your health
- poor concentration
- sleep disturbance, difficulty getting to sleep or waking early
- constant tiredness
- loss of interest in sex.

In depression, the levels of chemicals that transmit signals to the brain are abnormally low and treatment with antidepressants can bring them back to normal. These drugs are not addictive, unlike some tranquillisers, and you will be able to stop taking them once you have fully recovered from depression. Most people take them for three to six months.

The important thing about anxiety and depression is to realise that it is common and it can be helped. Often just discussing what you feel with someone else who has been through the same is enough. Many towns now have a self-help group attached to the rehab service which gives long-term support where this is needed. If you have any of the symptoms listed above, don't just struggle on waiting for them to go, consult your doctor.

KEY POINTS

After a heart attack:

- Most problems occur in the first 48 hours; after that life soon returns to normal

- Regular exercise can help you to make a full recovery, but it should be supervised

- Emotional problems after a heart attack are common and can be helped by talking about them and sometimes by drugs

Look after your heart

Is it too late?

You may think it is too late to think about prevention if you have already had a heart attack or developed angina. In fact, there is a lot you can do to reduce your chances of having another heart attack by reducing your risk factors. This is especially important after bypass surgery because it means that your new blood vessels will be less likely to fur up again.

Some diseases, notably diabetes and hypertension (raised blood pressure), can increase the risk of developing coronary heart disease (CHD), but this risk is reduced if the conditions are well controlled with suitable medication.

Lowering cholesterol

Lipids is the collective term used by doctors to refer to fat-like substances in the blood. Cholesterol is the best known, but another type, triglycerides, also play a role in CHD.

Cholesterol has a bad reputation as a cause of disease of the heart and blood vessels, but it also performs some essential functions in the body and no one could do without it entirely. It is manufactured in the liver and is used in the cell membranes, to make bile and to form vital chemical messengers (or hormones). Even if you excluded cholesterol completely from your diet, therefore, you would always have some in your blood.

In practice, most diets in western countries include large amounts of animal fat which the body converts into cholesterol. These fats are absorbed by the stomach and intestines and pass to the liver, where they are broken down and circulated to the rest of the body to provide energy or to be stored in the fat cells. The fat circulates through the body in the blood in tiny particles containing mixtures of cholesterol and other fats.

Measuring blood cholesterol
LDL and HDL
When you have a blood cholesterol measurement, the laboratory will usually measure several other fats as well. The total cholesterol level is made up of two main parts, called low-density lipoprotein (LDL) and high-density lipoprotein (HDL).

LDL is the 'bad' cholesterol which, when the level is too high, builds up in the arterial wall to produce atheroma. About two-thirds of the cholesterol in the blood is LDL, and this is usually what doctors are referring to when they say that you have a high cholesterol level.

HDL is, on the other hand, a 'good' cholesterol and, the higher the level, the less likely you are to get heart

Absorption and distribution of fat in the body

Fats are absorbed in the stomach and processed by the liver before being released into the circulation.

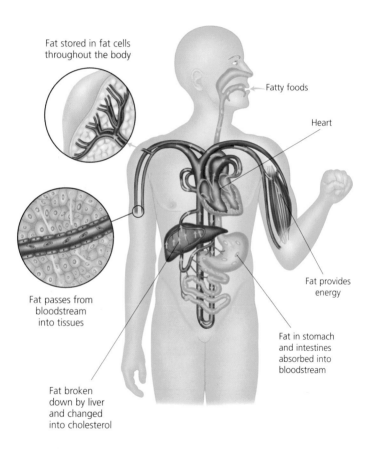

Fat stored in fat cells throughout the body

Fatty foods

Heart

Fat provides energy

Fat passes from bloodstream into tissues

Fat in stomach and intestines absorbed into bloodstream

Fat broken down by liver and changed into cholesterol

disease. Women have a higher HDL level than men but this difference usually disappears after the menopause. HDL levels are also increased if you take regular exercise.

Triglycerides

Triglycerides are the third type of fat measured in a blood sample. Triglycerides make up most of the fat in the fat cells of your body and, when released, provide the energy that you need for everyday activities. Although triglycerides are not found in any quantity in arterial walls, high levels of triglycerides in the blood are indirectly linked to CHD.

Most people who have angina or a heart attack have high lipid levels, which are partly the result of what they eat and partly genetic (running in families). By careful dieting we can reduce lipid or cholesterol levels by 10–20 per cent but, if we want to lower them more than this, drugs are usually necessary.

You may find that your doctor prescribes more than one drug to lower lipids, because they work in different ways. However, you will also be given advice on reducing the amount of cholesterol in your diet because this is necessary if the drug treatment is to be fully effective (see pages 104–6).

Statins

The big advance in the treatment of high cholesterol in the last 10 years has been the development of this new class of drug which works by slowing the production of cholesterol in the liver. Statins are able to lower cholesterol by up to 40 per cent and have very few side effects.

There have now been many important studies, involving thousands of patients in Europe, Australia and the USA, showing that this reduction in cholesterol is followed by a 20 to 30 per cent reduction in the risk of further heart attacks. The most common statins used at present are simvastatin and atorvastatin, although there are many more being developed.

These drugs are usually taken as a single dose in the evening and have few side effects. Very occasionally they may cause inflammation in the muscles of the arms and legs, an aching that feels like flu. This occurs in the first few weeks after starting treatment and should be reported immediately to your doctor. It settles once the tablets are stopped.

If you have no problems with these drugs in the first few weeks you are unlikely to develop any after that.

Fibrates

For some individuals, particularly those with diabetes, the problem with the lipids may be not so much with cholesterol as with triglycerides, when another group of drugs called the fibrates may be used. They too may produce muscular pains in the first few weeks but otherwise have few side effects. They can reduce cholesterol levels by 10 to 15 per cent and cut the risk of CHD by about the same percentage.

Ezetimibe

Ezetimibe acts by blocking the absorption of cholesterol in the gut and reduces cholesterol by about 15 per cent. It is taken once daily in tablet form, and is used in combination with a statin or in patients who are statin intolerant.

Drug treatment for raised cholesterol

Drug group	Examples of generic names	Example of trade names
statins	rosuvastatin	Crestor
	fluvastatin	Lescol
	atorvastatin	Lipitor
	pravastatin	Lipostat
	simvastatin	Zocor
fibrates	bezafibrate	Bezalip
	gemfibrozil	Lopid
resins	colestipol hydro-chloride	Colestid
	colestyramine	Questran
cholesterol-lowering drug	ezetimibe	Ezetrol

Resins

Resins reduce cholesterol levels by binding cholesterol in the intestines and affecting their absorption into the body. These are taken in the form of a powder, usually in fruit juice, once or twice a day. As they are not absorbed into the body, they cannot cause any serious side effects in body tissues, but they can cause flatulence and belching or constipation in some people.

Resins too have been shown to reduce the risk of further heart attack, but they are less potent than the statins and reduce the risk by only 10 to 15 per cent.

Improving your diet

Changing the sort of food that you have eaten all your life may not be easy but it is an important way to reduce the risk of further heart attack. The basic rules are fairly simple and given in the box on page 106.

Reduce your intake of animal and dairy fat

Eating healthily doesn't mean giving up everything you enjoy or eating nothing but 'rabbit food'. Most people in this country consume far more fat, and especially animal or dairy fat, than is good for them and cutting down would be a health bonus for your whole family.

Red meat, hard cheeses, butter, cream, full-fat milk and yoghurt as well as cooking fats like lard are all high in so-called saturated fats. It is wise to cut down on saturated fats or just keep these foods for special occasions.

Certain foods, such as eggs, liver, kidney and shellfish, contain fairly high levels of cholesterol. You should restrict these to some extent, although they probably contribute less to the level of blood cholesterol than foods high in animal fats.

In general, cutting down on fats is a good way to lose weight, and many people find that, after changing their diet, they also get much less indigestion. It's worth bearing in mind too that many processed and prepared foods such as pies, biscuits, cakes and so on may be high in animal fats. So, of course, are burgers!

Now that we are all starting to become more health conscious, many foods in supermarkets are labelled to give us some idea of the fat content.

Healthy eating

A high-fibre diet rich in fruit and vegetables wil benefit your overall health.

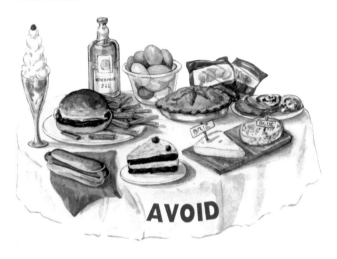

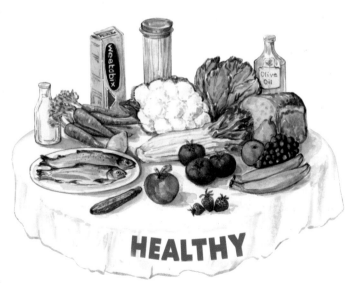

Polyunsaturated fats

As well as reducing the overall amount of fat in your diet, you should try to use polyunsaturated fats – generally those from vegetable sources which are liquid at room temperature – or monounsaturated fat, like olive oil, whenever you can. If you are not sure which are the healthy oils, check the label or ask a dietitian as one or two vegetable oils are not good for the heart. Coconut oil in particular is almost as bad for the heart as pork dripping!

Fruit and vegetables

The other major change that will improve your diet from a health viewpoint is to eat as many pieces of fruit and vegetables as you can – at least five portions every day. If you can also increase your intake of other fibre-rich foods such as wholemeal bread, brown rice and pasta and breakfast cereals, especially oats, you will be well on the way to a diet that's good for your overall health as well as your heart.

Fortunately the food industry is beginning to realise the importance of a healthy diet, and there are now

---

Four steps to healthy eating

Anyone can eat more healthily by following these simple guidelines:

- Cut down the total amount of fat in your diet
- Replace animal fats (dairy fats) with vegetable oils, especially olive oil
- Eat more fresh fruit and vegetables
- Go on a sensible weight-reducing diet if necessary

many good recipe books to help. What many writers ignore, however, is the higher cost of some healthy foods, and this often puts a strain on the family budget. If this is a real problem you should discuss the matter with your doctor. There may be benefits that you are entitled to, or a dietitian may be able to advise on the best way to budget the weekly shopping.

Smoking

The benefits of stopping smoking are real and start from the day that you give up and, after five years your risk of having another heart attack will be halved. You do have to stop completely, however: cutting down or changing from cigarettes to cigars or a pipe does little to reduce the risk.

Many people find it easy to stop smoking in hospital, but it's much harder to keep it up when you go home. If you have smoked since you were a teenager it can be a real problem. This is where all the family can help, because there is nothing worse, when the craving is there, than for your partner or daughter to light up. Hospitals are now 'no smoking' areas and your home should be too!

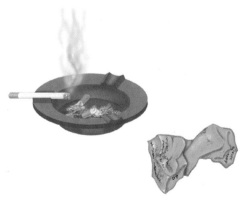

What is the best way of giving up? That's going to be different for everyone. Some people have found it easiest to stop suddenly. Others prefer to stop gradually, perhaps cutting down by a cigarette a day over several weeks. Part of the problem is an addiction to nicotine itself, and for some the use of nicotine chewing gum or skin patches can be a great help.

Sometimes talking to others trying to give up is the best help, and many hospitals and health centres run 'stopping smoking' sessions. Some even swear by hypnosis – as doctors we don't care so long as you kick the habit!

One of the things that often puts people off giving up smoking is the tendency to put on weight afterwards. We are still not sure why this happens. Certainly the appetite improves, and some people take to eating sweets to reduce their craving for a cigarette. On average most people put on between half and one stone in the first six months after stopping smoking. However, if you change to a healthier, low-fat diet at the same time the extra weight usually comes off again gradually over the next six to twelve months.

A new drug bupropion (Zyban) has received a great deal of publicity because it can be very effective in helping patients to give up smoking. It is not suitable for everyone, however; consult your doctor if you think that it could help you.

Stress

When you develop angina or have had a heart attack, it is a real opportunity to weigh up the priorities in your life. You may feel that a job that has occupied a large proportion of your time and energy over the years now seems less important than your family and friends and your other interests. Although there is no scientific proof that changing the way that you live reduces your risk, it will certainly improve the quality of your life.

Protective factors
Alcohol
There has been quite a lot of publicity about the good effects of alcohol when taken in moderation. Of course, high levels of alcohol taken on a regular basis can poison the heart as well as other internal organs such as the brain and the liver.

So what is moderation? The amount of alcohol that seems to be good for you is around two to three units a day, with women sticking to the lower end of the range. A unit is a measure of spirits, a small glass of wine or half a pint of beer or cider. Although it was first thought that red wine was particularly good at preventing heart attacks, it now seems that any form of alcohol has the same effect.

Exercise
Regular exercise is also good for you and can protect against CHD. There have been many studies in the USA and Europe which show that, if you take regular exercise (20 minutes two or three times a week), this reduces the risk of CHD when compared with those who don't.

If you've actually had a heart attack, you will be taught about exercise in your rehabilitation sessions. In fact anyone who has any form of CHD may well benefit from exercise too. If you have never exercised before and are unsure how to start, do ask your doctor's advice.

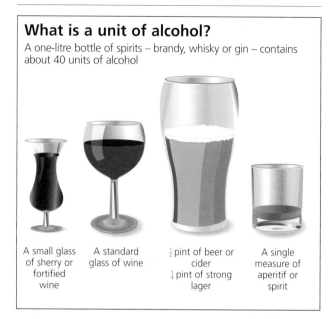

What is a unit of alcohol?

A one-litre bottle of spirits – brandy, whisky or gin – contains about 40 units of alcohol

A small glass of sherry or fortified wine

A standard glass of wine

½ pint of beer or cider
¼ pint of strong lager

A single measure of aperitif or spirit

What type of exercise you go for is probably not important, provided that it stimulates the heart and circulation sufficiently. You should do what you like best: walking, swimming, jogging, exercising in the gym and even dancing are all likely to help. Most people will need to start relatively slowly and build up to longer and more strenuous sessions gradually. If you go to a gym or an exercise class, you should be shown how to warm up properly before and afterwards, and it's a good idea to get into the habit of doing this with any exercise session.

The idea of 'going for the burn'– exercising until it hurts and beyond – has been thoroughly discredited. If you feel pain, dizziness or find it hard to breathe, stop and rest. And always have a break from exercise if you are injured or not feeling well.

What should you weigh?

- The body mass index (BMI) is a useful measure of healthy weight
- Find out your height in metres and weight in kilograms
- Calculate your BMI like this

$$BMI = \frac{Your\ weight\ (kg)}{[Your\ height\ (metres)\ x\ Your\ height\ (metres)]}$$

$$e.g.\ 24.8 = \frac{70}{[1.68\ x\ 1.68]}$$

- You are recommended to try to maintain a BMI in the range 20–25
- The chart below is an easier way of estimating your BMI. Read off your height and your weight. The point where the lines cross in the chart indicates your BMI

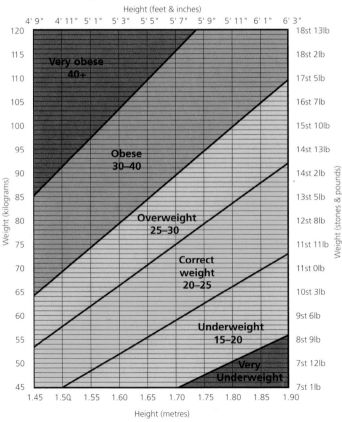

Working with your doctor

Although smoking and exercise levels are major risk factors that are to a large extent under your own control, there are other spheres where you and your doctor will need to work together to minimise the risk of further problems. People with conditions that make CHD more likely, such as diabetes and hypertension (high blood pressure), need to try to keep these under good control by regular checks at the surgery.

Hypertension

Make a big effort to take your tablets regularly, even though you have no symptoms. See your doctor for regular blood pressure checks.

Diabetes

Try to keep your weight as close as possible to what it should be for your height.

Do your best to keep your blood glucose levels within the normal range by paying careful attention to your diet and taking your prescribed treatment properly. Exercise is important because it helps to reduce your weight and also reduces your insulin requirement. Blood pressure control is particularly important in people with diabetes.

Raised lipid levels

Make an effort to stick to your diet, take any tablets correctly and attend for regular blood tests.

What to do in an emergency

A heart attack can happen anywhere; everyone should know what to do to help someone if they collapse and the heart stops beating. Basic life support (BLS) is not difficult and it may be literally life saving to learn how to do it.

Instructors are available in most towns, from voluntary agencies such as St John Ambulance or from the local hospital. If you or someone with you develops chest pain that seems similar to the heart pain associated with an earlier heart attack, there are some basic steps to follow:

- Rest, sitting or lying down
- Take GTN medicine and wait for five minutes
- If the pain is still as bad or worse after five to ten minutes, take a second dose
- If this has no effect, telephone for an ambulance
- Chew on an aspirin (unless you or the person concerned is known to be allergic to it) as this will start to thin the blood and discourage clots.

WHAT TO DO IN AN EMERGENCY – ABC

Airway: ensure that there is nothing preventing air getting in through the nose and mouth.
Breathing: see whether there is any spontaneous breathing.
Circulation: feel for a pulse in the neck.

If there is no breathing and you can't feel the pulse, a cardiac arrest has probably occurred. Call for help and, if you know how, start mouth-to-mouth respiration and cardiac massage.

KEY POINTS

- Changing to a healthy diet improves your fitness and helps your heart

- Drug treatment to lower cholesterol reduces the risk of CHD

- Stopping smoking reduces your risk further and is effective immediately

- Regular exercise improves the state of your heart and circulation

Useful addresses

We have included the following organisations because, on preliminary investigation, they may be of use to the reader. However, we do not have first-hand experience of each organisation and so cannot guarantee the organisation's integrity. The reader must therefore exercise his or her own discretion and judgement when making further enquiries.

Benefits Enquiry Line
Tel: 0800 882200
Minicom: 0800 243355
Website: www.dwp.gov.uk
N. Ireland: 0800 220674

Government agency giving information and advice on sickness and disability benefits for people with disabilities and their carers.

Blood Pressure Association

60 Cranmer Terrace
London SW17 0QS
Tel: 020 8772 4994
Fax: 020 8772 4999
Email: info@bpassoc.org.uk
Website: www.bpassoc.org.uk

Raises public awareness about, and offers information and support to, people affected by high blood pressure and health-care professionals. Has a wide selection of literature and free membership scheme.

British Heart Foundation

14 Fitzhardinge Street
London W1H 6DH
Tel: 020 7935 0185
Fax: 020 7486 5820
Helpline: 0845 070 8070
Website: www.bhf.org.uk

Funds research, promotes education and raises money to buy equipment to treat heart disease. Information and support available for people with heart conditions. Via Heartstart UK, arranges training in emergency life-saving techniques for lay people. Publications orderline 01604 640016; local groups 020 7487 7110.

British Hypertension Society Information Service

Clinical Sciences Building, Level 5, Leicester Royal Infirmary
PO Box 65, Leicester LE2 7LX
Tel: 07717 467973
Email: bhs@le.ac.uk
Website: www.bhsoc.org

Provides information to doctors, nurses, and other health professionals who work in the field of hypertension and cardiovascular disease. Has no patient leaflets; however, maintains a list of blood pressure monitors that is available to the public on request. This list is also on the website.

Cardiomyopathy Association
40 The Metro Centre, Tolpits Lane
Watford, Herts WD18 9SB
Tel: 01923 249977
Fax: 01923 249987
Helpline: 0800 018 1024
Email: info@cardiomyopathy.org
Website: www.cardiomyopathy.org

Support organisation helping patients and medical professionals with information on hypertrophic, dilated and other forms of cardiomyopathy.

Chest, Heart and Stroke Scotland
65 North Castle Street
Edinburgh EH2 3LT
Tel: 0131 225 6963
Fax: 0131 220 6313
Helpline: 0845 077 6000
Email: admin@chss.org.uk
Website: www.chss.org.uk

Aims to improve the quality of life for people in Scotland affected by chest, heart and stroke illness through medical research, advice and information, and support in the community.

Chest, Heart and Stroke, Northern Ireland

22 Great Victoria Street
Belfast BT2 7LX
Tel: 028 9032 0184
Fax: 028 9033 3487
Email: mail@nichsa.com
Helpline: 0845 769 7299
Website: www.nichsa.com

Aims to promote the prevention of, and alleviate the suffering resulting from, chest, heart and stroke illnesses in Northern Ireland through advice and information.

Diabetes UK

Macleod House, 10 Parkway
London NW1 7AA
Tel: 020 7424 1000
Fax: 020 7424 1001
Helpline: 0845 120 2960
Email: info@diabetes.org.uk
Website: www.diabetes.org.uk

Provides advice and information for people with diabetes and their families. Helpline operates a translation service. Has local support groups.

Heart UK

7 North Road
Maidenhead, Berks SL6 1PE
Tel: 01628 628638
Fax: 01628 628698
Email: ask@heartuk.org.uk
Website: www.heartuk.org.uk

Offers information, advice and support to people with coronary heart disease and especially those at high risk of familial hypercholesterolaemia. Members receive bi-monthly magazine.

Lifesavers, The Royal Life Saving Society UK

River House, High Street
Broom, Warwicks B50 4HN
Tel: 01789 773994
Fax: 01789 773995
Email: lifesavers@rlss.org.uk
Website: www.lifesavers.org.uk

Runs courses throughout the UK in water safety, rescue techniques and life support.

MedicAlert

1 Bridge Wharf, 156 Caledonian Road
London N1 9UU
Tel: 020 7833 3034
Fax: 020 7278 0647
Infoline: 0800 581420
Email: info@medicalert.org.uk
Website: www.medicalert.org.uk

Provides emergency identification with body-worn jewellery for people with hidden medical conditions. The 24-hour emergency telephone service accepts reverse charge calls; can access personal details from anywhere in the world in over 100 languages.

NHS Direct

Freephone: 0845 4647 (24 hours)

Trained operatives will assess symptoms and give advice on the level of care needed, as well as provide general information.

National Institute for Health and Clinical Excellence (NICE)
MidCity Place, 71 High Holborn
London WC1V 6NA
Tel: 020 7067 5800
Fax: 020 7067 5801
Email: nice@nice.nhs.uk
Website: www.nice.org.uk

Provides national guidance on the promotion of good health and the prevention and treatment of ill-health. Patient information leaflets are available for each piece of guidance issued.

Prodigy Website
Sowerby Centre for Health Informatics at Newcastle (SCHIN), Bede House, All Saints Business Centre
Newcastle upon Tyne NE1 2ES
Tel: 0191 243 6100
Fax: 0191 243 6101
Email: prodigy-enquiries@schin.co.uk
Website: www.prodigy.nhs.uk/PILS/indexself.asp

A website mainly for GPs giving information for patients listed by disease plus named self-help organisations.

Quit (Smoking Quitlines)
211 Old Street
London EC1V 9NR
Tel: 020 7251 1551

Fax: 020 7251 1661
Helpline: 0800 002200
Scotland: 0800 848484
Wales: 0800 169 0169 (NHS helpline)
Email: info@quit.org.uk
Website: www.quit.org.uk

Offers advice on giving up smoking in English and
Asian languages, and also to schools and on
pregnancy. Runs training courses for health
professionals. Can put people in touch with local
support groups. Has free same-day advice on email:
stopsmoking@quit.org.uk

Resuscitation Council (UK)
5th Floor, Tavistock House North, Tavistock Square
London WC1H 9HR
Tel: 020 7388 4678
Fax: 020 7383 0773
Email: enquiries@resus.org.uk
Website: www.resus.org.uk

Sets standards and runs courses for health-care
professionals. Sells publications on resuscitation and
funds research.

St John Ambulance
27 St John's Lane
London EC1M 4BU
Tel: 020 7324 4000
Fax: 0870 010 4065
Helpline: 0870 010 4950 (office hours)
Email: info@nhq.sja.org.uk
Website: www.sja.org.uk

Provides training locally throughout the UK and first aid at public events via its members. Offers a variety of welfare services in local communities.

The internet as a source of further information

After reading this book, you may feel that you would like further information on the subject. The internet is of course an excellent place to look and there are many websites with useful information about medical disorders, related charities and support groups.

For those who do not have a computer at home some bars and cafes offer facilities for accessing the internet. These are listed in the *Yellow Pages* under 'Internet Bars and Cafes' and 'Internet Providers'. Your local library offers a similar facility and has staff to help you find the information that you need.

It should always be remembered, however, that the internet is unregulated and anyone is free to set up a website and add information to it. Many websites offer impartial advice and information that have been compiled and checked by qualified medical professionals. Some, on the other hand, are run by commercial organisations with the purpose of promoting their own products. Others still are run by pressure groups, some of which will provide carefully assessed and accurate information whereas others may be suggesting medications or treatments that are not supported by the medical and scientific community.

Unless you know the address of the website you want to visit – for example, www.familydoctor.co.uk – you may find the following guidelines useful when searching the internet for information.

Search engines and other searchable sites

Google (www.google.co.uk) is the most popular search engine used in the UK, followed by Yahoo! (http://uk.yahoo.com) and MSN (www.msn.co.uk). Also popular are the search engines provided by Internet Service Providers such as Tiscali and other sites such as the BBC site (www.bbc.co.uk).

In addition to the search engines that index the whole web, there are also medical sites with search facilities, which act almost like mini-search engines, but cover only medical topics or even a particular area of medicine. Again, it is wise to look at who is responsible for compiling the information offered to ensure that it is impartial and medically accurate. The NHS Direct site (www.nhsdirect.nhs.uk) is an example of a searchable medical site.

Links to many British medical charities can be found at the Association of Medical Research Charities' website (www.amrc.org.uk) and at Charity Choice (www.charitychoice.co.uk).

Search phrases

Be specific when entering a search phrase. Searching for information on 'cancer' will return results for many different types of cancer as well as on cancer in general. You may even find sites offering astrological information. More useful results will be returned by using search phrases such as 'lung cancer' and 'treatments for lung cancer'. Both Google and Yahoo! offer an advanced search option that includes the ability to search for the exact phrase; enclosing the search phrase in quotes, that is, 'treatments for lung cancer', will have the same effect. Limiting a search to an exact phrase reduces the number of results returned but it is best to refine a search to an exact match only if you are not getting useful results with a normal search. Adding 'UK' to your search term will bring up mainly British sites, so a good phrase might be 'lung cancer' UK (don't include UK within the quotes).

Always remember that the internet is international and unregulated. It holds a wealth of valuable information but individual sites may be biased, out of date or just plain wrong. Family Doctor Publications accepts no responsibility for the content of links published in this series.

Index

ABC of emergency treatment
113

ACE (angiotensin-converting
enzyme) inhibitors 27,
72, 88–9, 90

acebutolol 88

activity, resumption after
heart attack 86

adenosine, use in radioactive
isotope tests 59

adrenaline (epinephrine) 69

affluence, association with
coronary heart disease
5, 7

African–Caribbean origin 41

age, and risk of CHD 34–5

alcohol consumption 109
– units of alcohol 110

amlodipine 88

aneurysms 19, 20

angina 2, 18, 27, 32, 45,
53, 65
– after a heart attack 87
– case history 30
– cause 1
– exercise ECG 56–7
– medical treatments
65–6, 72, 80, 88–9
– aspirin 71
– beta blockers 69
– calcium channel
blockers 69, 71
– clopidogrel 71
– nicorandil 71
– nitrates 66–8, 70
– narrowed coronary
arteries 48
– surgical treatments 72,
80
– angioplasty 73–5
– bypass surgery (CABG)
75–9
– symptoms 46
– unstable angina 21,
46–7, 71

angiograms 61–3

angioplasty 10, 21, 73–5, 80
– clopidogrel treatment 71

angiotensin **90**

ankles, swollen **27, 29, 53, 89**

anterior descending coronary artery **16, 17**

anti-platelet drugs **88–9**

anticoagulants **21**

antidepressants **96**

anxiety **95, 96**

aorta, aortic arch **15, 16, 17**

aortic aneurysm **19, 20**

aortic valve **15**

arms, pain in **46, 47**

arrhythmias **3, 25, 27, 85**

arteries **13**
 – hardening of *see* atheroma

aspirin **10, 22, 66, 71, 87**
 – benefits after heart attack **82, 113**

Association of Medical Research Charities **123**

asthma **52**
 – and beta blockers **69, 90**

atenolol **30, 88–9**
 – *see also* beta blockers

atheroma (atherosclerosis) **18–19, 36**
 – clinical effects **20**
 – and high blood pressure **43**
 – thrombosis **21–2**
 – which arteries are affected **19, 21**

atorvastatin **88–9, 102, 103**

atria (auricles) **12, 15**

atrial fibrillation **27**

automatic blood pressure machines **42**

balloon angioplasty *see* angioplasty

basic life support (BLS) **112–13**

bed rest **92**

Benefits Enquiry Line **115**

beta blockers **10, 27, 80, 88–9**
 – use after heart attack **90**
 – use in angina **69**

bezafibrate (Bezalip) **103**

bisoprolol **88–9**

black American people **41**

blood circulation **12, 14, 16**

blood clots *see* thrombosis

blood pressure **40**
 – effect of beta blockers **69**
 – in heart attack **25**
 – measurement **41, 42**
 – *see also* high blood pressure

Blood Pressure Association **116**

blood supply of heart **16–17**
 – *see also* coronary arteries

blood thinning medication **71, 88–9**

blood vessels
 – effect of smoking **37**
 – *see also* arteries; coronary arteries; veins

body mass index (BMI) **111**

breathlessness **3, 27, 28, 52–3**

British Heart Foundation **116**

British Hypertension Society Information Service **116–17**

bronchitis **52**
 – and beta blockers **69, 90**

buccal nitrate **68**
bupropion (Zyban) **108**
'burn-out' **39–40**
bypass surgery (CABG, coronary artery bypass graft) **10, 21, 75–9, 80**

calcium channel blockers (calcium antagonists) **69, 71, 80, 88–9**
cannulas **81**
capillaries **13**
captopril **88–9**
cardiac arrest **25, 113**
cardiac care units (CCUs) **25, 84–5**
cardiac rehabilitation **92–3, 109**
cardiomyopathies **3**
Cardiomyopathy Association **117**
cardiovascular system **13**
carvedilol **88–9**
case histories
 – angina **30**
 – heart attack **31**
catheter for coronary angiography **61**
causes of coronary heart disease **1, 8, 10**
Charity Choice **123**
check-ups **35**
Chest, Heart and Stroke **117–18**
chest pain **45–6**
 – in angina **46**
 – associated with palpitations **52**
 – caused by trapped nerves **51, 52**
 – from muscles **50, 51**
 – in heart attack **22, 47, 49**
 – in indigestion **49, 51**
 – in pleurisy **50, 51**
 – in shingles **50, 51**
 – in unstable angina **46–7**
 – in viral infections **50, 51**
cholesterol **34, 36–7, 98–9**
 – blood levels in diabetes **44**
 – in diet **104**
 – Framingham study **38**
 – LDL-cholesterol **18**
 – measurement of blood levels **99**
 – raised blood levels **112**
cholesterol-lowering drugs **10, 66, 88–9, 101–3**
chronic bronchitis **52**
cigarettes *see* smoking
cilazapril **88–9**
circulation of blood **12, 14, 16**
circumflex branch, left coronary artery **16, 17**
clopidogrel **71, 87, 88–9**
'clot-buster' drugs (thrombolytics) **10, 22, 81–4**
clotting of blood **21**
coconut oil **106**
coffee, as cause of palpitations **52**
cold hands and feet **69, 89**
cold weather, effect on angina **46**
colestipol hydrochloride (Colestid) **103**
colestyramine (Questran) **103**

collateral circulation **25, 26, 30**

congenital heart disease **3**

constipation **89, 103**

coronary angiography **61–3, 64**

coronary arteries **1, 16–17, 32**
 – effect of nitrates **67**
 – what happens in CHD **18**

coronary artery disease (CAD) **2**

coronary heart disease (CHD) **1, 20, 32**
 – as cause of death **4, 5, 6, 9**
 – causes **8, 10**
 – new treatments **10**
 – one-, two- or three-vessel disease **19, 21**
 – risk factors **33–44**
 – stages **48**
 – what happens with time **27, 30**
 – what happens to the coronary arteries **18**
 – when it was first recognised **7**
 – who gets it **5–7**

coronary thrombosis **2, 23, 24**
 – *see also* heart attack

cough **53**
 – as side effect of medication **89**

Crestor (rosuvastatin) **88–9, 103**

death, causes of **4**

death rates from coronary heart disease **9**

defibrillators **84, 85**

deoxygenated blood **12, 14**

depression **95–6**

diabetes **34, 38, 43–4, 98, 112**
 – symptoms of heart attack **49**

Diabetes UK **118**

diagnosis **54, 64**
 – coronary angiography **61–3**
 – echocardiography **59–60**
 – heart tracing (ECG) **55–7**
 – radioactive isotope tests **57–9**
 – use of nitrates **66, 68**

diastolic pressure **41**

diet **7, 8, 10, 36–7**
 – fats and cholesterol **99**
 – improving it **104–7**

digoxin **27**

diltiazem **88–9**

dipyridamole, use in radioactive isotope tests **59**

diuretics **27**

dizziness, as side effect of medication **66, 89**

dobutamine, use in radioactive isotope tests **59**

driving after a heart attack **93**

drug treatments
 – after heart attack **87–90**
 – for angina **65–72, 80**
 – lipid-lowering **101–3**

dye tests (coronary angiography) **61–3**

ECG (electrocardiograph) **55–7, 64, 81**

echocardiography **59–60, 64**
electric shock treatment (defibrillation) **84, 85**
emergencies, what to do **112–13**
emphysema **52**
enalapril **88–9**
epinephrine (adrenaline) **69**
exercise
– benefits **25, 109–10, 112**
– lack of **8, 34**
– pain during see angina; unstable angina
exercise ECG **56–7**
exercise programmes **93**
ezetimibe (Ezetrol) **102, 103**

faintness **25**
– associated with palpitations **52**
familial hyperlipidaemia (FH) **36**
family history of CHD **31, 34, 35, 36**
fat deposits see atheroma
fats
– absorption and distribution **100**
– in blood see cholesterol; triglycerides
– in diet **36–7**
– improving your diet **104, 106**
fibrates **102**
first aid **112–13**
flatulence, as side effect of medication **103**
fluid retention **3, 27, 28–9**
fluvastatin **88–9**
fosinopril **88–9**

Framingham study **38**
fruit and vegetables **106–7**

gangrene **19, 20**
gemfibrozil (Lopid) **103**
gender differences in CHD **34–5**
generic names of drugs **89**
genetic factors in CHD **34, 35, 36**
glyceryl trinitrate (GTN) **65, 66–8, 87, 88–9, 90**
– taking it in an emergency **113**
gullet, pain from **49**

HDL (high-density lipoprotein)-cholesterol **99, 101**
headache, as side effect of medication **66, 89**
healthy eating **104–7**
heart
– blood supply **16–17**
– effect of high blood pressure **43**
– effect of nitrates **67**
– structure and function **12, 14–16**
heart attack **3, 18, 19, 30, 32, 36, 45, 53**
– case history **31**
– cause **1**
– as complication of angiography **61**
– coronary thrombosis **21–2, 23, 48**
– driving **93–4**
– duration of hospital stay **85–6**

heart attack (contd)
- going on holiday **94–5**
- recovery period **85–7**
- rehabilitation **92–3**
- relationship to stress **39**
- returning to work **94**
- sexual activity **94**
- symptoms **47, 49**
- treatment **87–91**
  - emergency assistance **81, 112–13**
  - regulating the heart beat **84–5**
  - thrombolytics ('clot busters') **81–4**
- treatment priorities **82**
- what happens **22–5**
- what to do in an emergency **112–13**
heart failure **3, 25, 27, 45**
- breathlessness **28, 52**
- swollen ankles **29**
heart rhythm irregularities (arrhythmias) **3, 25, 27, 52, 85**
heart tracing (ECG) **55–7**
Heart UK **118–19**
'heartburn' **49**
help, where to find it
- searching the internet **122–4**
- useful addresses **115–22**
high blood pressure **27, 34, 38, 40–1, 98, 112**
- Blood Pressure Association **116**
- British Hypertension Society Information Service **116–17**
- how common it is **41–3**
- why it is bad **43**
holidays after heart attack **94–5**
home, returning after a heart attack **86–7**
HRT (hormone replacement therapy) **35**
hypertension *see* high blood pressure

impotence **69**
indigestion **49, 51, 53**
- as side effect of medication **71, 89**
insulin **43**
internal mammary artery grafts **77**
ischaemic heart disease (IHD) **2**
isosorbide dinitrate/ mononitrate **88–9**
isotope scans **57–9, 64**

jaw pain **46, 47**

'laid-back' personality type **40**
LDL (low-density lipoprotein)-cholesterol **18, 99**
left coronary artery **16, 17**
legs
- aching muscles **69**
- swollen **27, 29, 53**
Lifesavers, The Royal Lifesaving Society UK **119**
lifestyle, role in coronary heart disease **5, 7**
lifestyle adjustments **66, 86**
lipids **98**

– raised blood levels **112**
– *see also* cholesterol
Lipitor (atorvastatin) **88–9,
102, 103**
Lipostat (pravastatin) **88–9,
103**
lisinopril **88–9**
Lopid (gemfibrozil) **103**
lungs
– fluid retention **28**
– gas exchange **13**

medical help, when to seek it
68, 87, 113
MedicAlert **119**
menopause, effect on risk of
CHD **34–5**
metoprolol **88–9**
mitral valve **15**
modifiable risk factors **33, 34**
monitoring of heart beat **25**
monounsaturated fats **106**
morphine **81**
muscle pain **50, 51**
– as side effect of
medication **102**
myocardial infarction (MI) **2**
– *see also* heart attack
myocardium **22**

National Institute for Health
and Clinical Excellence
(NICE) **120**
nausea **25, 47**
neck pain **46**
NHS Direct **119–20**
nicardipine **88–9**
nicorandil **71, 88–9**
nicotine replacement therapy
108

nifedipine **88–9**
night-time symptoms
– breathlessness **52**
– chest pain **47**
nightmares **89**
nitrates **65, 66–8, 80, 88–9,
90**
– ways of taking them **70**
– *see also* glyceryl trinitrate
(GTN)
non-modifiable risk factors
33, 34

obesity **10, 34**
– risk of diabetes **43**
oesophagus, pain from **49**
oils **106**
one-vessel disease **19, 21**
osteoporosis **35, 52**
oxygen treatment **81**
oxygenated blood **12, 14**

pain *see* chest pain
palpitations **3, 52**
paramedics **81, 82**
PCI *see* angioplasty
pentaerythritol tetranitrate
88–9
perindopril **88–9**
personality, effect on CHD
risk **39–40**
physiotherapists **93**
pipe smokers **38**
– *see also* smoking
plaques **18, 19, 36**
platelets **21**
– effect of aspirin **87**
– effect of smoking **37**
pleurisy **50, 51**
pneumonia **50**

polyunsaturated fats **106**
potassium channel activators
 88–9
poverty **8**
pravastatin **88–9, 103**
prevention **98**
 – improving your diet
 104–7
 – lowering cholesterol
 98–103
 – priorities **108–9**
 – protective factors
 109–10
 – stopping smoking **107–8**
processed food **104**
Prodigy Website **120**
propranolol **88–9**
proprietary names of drugs **88**
pulmonary arteries **17**
pulmonary valve **15**

Questran (colestyramine)
 103
quinapril **88–9**
Quit (Smoking Quitlines)
 120–1

radioactive isotope tests
 57–9, 64
ramipril **88–9**
red wine consumption **109**
regional variations in
 coronary heart disease
 6, 7, 8
rehabilitation after heart
 attack **92–3, 109**
resins **103**
resting ECG **55–6**
Resuscitation Council (UK)
 121

risk factors for CHD **33–4, 44**
 – age and gender **34–5**
 – diabetes **43–4**
 – diet and cholesterol
 36–7
 – family history **31, 35**
 – high blood pressure
 40–3
 – smoking **37–8**
 – stress **38–40**
rosuvastatin **88–9, 103**

St John Ambulance **121–2**
saturated fats **104**
scarring of heart muscle **25,
 27, 32, 86**
sexual activity, resumption
 after heart attack **94**
sexual problems **69**
shingles **50**
side effects of medication
 66, 89
 – of aspirin **71**
 – of beta blockers **69**
 – of fibrates **102**
 – of nitrates **66**
 – of statins **102**
simvastatin **88–9, 102, 103**
size of heart attack **22, 25**
skin patches, nitrates **68, 70**
smoking **8, 10, 34, 37–8**
 – as cause of palpitations
 52
 – giving it up **107–8**
 – Quit (Smoking Quitlines)
 120–1
social deprivation **8**
statins **66, 88–9, 90, 101–2,
 103**
stents **10, 73, 74**

stomach pains **53**
streptokinase **82, 84**
  – *see also* thrombolytics
stress **34, 38–40, 108–9**
  – as cause of palpitations
    52
stress echocardiography
    59–60
stroke **19, 20**
  – as complication of
    angiography **61**
surgery **10, 21, 80**
  – angioplasty **73–5**
  – bypass surgery (CABG)
    75–9
sweating **25, 47**
swelling of ankles **27, 29,
    53, 89**
symptoms **45**
  – of angina **46**
  – breathlessness **52–3**
  – of depression **96**
  – of heart attack **47, 49**
  – of indigestion
    ('heartburn') **49, 51**
  – of muscle pain **50**
  – palpitations **52**
  – of pleurisy **50, 51**
  – of shingles **50, 51**
  – of trapped nerves **51, 52**
  – of unstable angina **46–7**
  – *see also* chest pain
systolic pressure **41**

tea, as cause of palpitations
    52
technetium scans **57–9**
tests **64**
  – coronary angiography
    61–3

  – echocardiography **59–60**
  – heart tracing (ECG) **55–7**
  – radioactive isotope tests
    57–9
thallium scans **57–9**
three-vessel disease **19, 21**
thrombolytics ('clot buster'
    drugs) **10, 22, 81–4**
thrombosis **21–2, 23, 24**
  – increased risk in smokers
    37
  – preventive medication **71**
tiredness **69, 89**
tPa (tissue plasminogen
    activator) **82, 84**
  – *see also* thrombolytics
trandolapril **88–9**
transducer **60**
trapped nerves **51, 52**
travel after heart attack
    94–5
treadmill test **56–7, 59, 64**
tricuspid valve **15**
triglyceride-lowering drugs
    102, 103
triglycerides **98, 101**
two-vessel disease **19, 21**

unstable angina **21, 46–7, 65**
  – drug treatment **71**

valves of heart **15**
valvular heart disease **3**
veins **13**
  – use for bypass surgery
    75–6
vena cavae **16**
ventricles **12, 15**
  – blood supply **16, 17**
verapamil **88**

viral infections, as cause of
  chest pain **50, 51**
vomiting **47**

'**w**ater tablets' (diuretics) **27**
weight
  – effect of stopping
    smoking **108**
  – what you should weigh
    111
weight reduction **104**

women, risk of CHD **34–5**
  – effect of diabetes **44**
work, returning after heart
    attack **94**

X-rays, angiograms **61–3, 64**

Zocor (simvastatin) **88–9,
    102, 103**
Zyban (bupropion) **108**

Your pages

We have included the following pages because they may help you manage your illness or condition and its treatment.

Before an appointment with a health professional, it can be useful to write down a short list of questions of things that you do not understand, so that you can make sure that you do not forget anything.

Some of the sections may not be relevant to your circumstances.

We are always pleased to receive constructive criticism or suggestions about how to improve the books. You can contact us at:

Email: familydoctor@btinternet.com
Letter: Family Doctor Publications
        PO Box 4664
        Poole
        BH15 1NN

Thank you

Health-care contact details

Name:

Job title:

Place of work:

Tel:

Name:

Job title:

Place of work:

Tel:

Name:

Job title:

Place of work:

Tel:

Name:

Job title:

Place of work:

Tel:

Significant past health events – illnesses/ operations/investigations/treatments

Event	Month	Year	Age (at time)

Appointments for health care

Name:

Place:

Date:

Time:

Tel:

Name:

Place:

Date:

Time:

Tel:

Name:

Place:

Date:

Time:

Tel:

Name:

Place:

Date:

Time:

Tel:

Appointments for health care

Name:

Place:

Date:

Time:

Tel:

Name:

Place:

Date:

Time:

Tel:

Name:

Place:

Date:

Time:

Tel:

Name:

Place:

Date:

Time:

Tel:

Current medication(s) prescribed by your doctor

Medicine name:

Purpose:

Frequency & dose:

Start date:

End date:

Medicine name:

Purpose:

Frequency & dose:

Start date:

End date:

Medicine name:

Purpose:

Frequency & dose:

Start date:

End date:

Medicine name:

Purpose:

Frequency & dose:

Start date:

End date:

Other medicines/supplements you are taking, not prescribed by your doctor

Medicine/treatment:

Purpose:

Frequency & dose:

Start date:

End date:

Medicine/treatment:

Purpose:

Frequency & dose:

Start date:

End date:

Medicine/treatment:

Purpose:

Frequency & dose:

Start date:

End date:

Medicine/treatment:

Purpose:

Frequency & dose:

Start date:

End date:

Questions to ask at appointments

(Note: do bear in mind that doctors work under great time
pressure, so long lists may not be helpful for either of you)

Questions to ask at appointments
(Note: do bear in mind that doctors work under great time pressure, so long lists may not be helpful for either of you)

Notes